AF689020

Fundamentals of Complementary and Alternative Medicine

Fundamentals of Complementary and Alternative Medicine

Ava Smith

SYRAWOOD PUBLISHING HOUSE
New York

Published by Syrawood Publishing House,
750 Third Avenue, 9th Floor,
New York, NY 10017, USA
www.syrawoodpublishinghouse.com

Fundamentals of Complementary and Alternative Medicine
Ava Smith

© 2022 Syrawood Publishing House

International Standard Book Number: 978-1-64740-104-7 (Hardback)

This book contains information obtained from authentic and highly regarded sources. All chapters are published with permission under the Creative Commons Attribution Share Alike License or equivalent. A wide variety of references are listed. Permissions and sources are indicated; for detailed attributions, please refer to the permissions page. Reasonable efforts have been made to publish reliable data and information, but the authors, editors and publisher cannot assume any responsibility for the validity of all materials or the consequences of their use.

Trademark Notice: Registered trademark of products or corporate names are used only for explanation and identification without intent to infringe.

Cataloging-in-Publication Data

Fundamentals of complementary and alternative medicine / Ava Smith.
p. cm.
Includes bibliographical references and index.
ISBN 978-1-64740-104-7
1. Alternative medicine. 2. Medicine. 3. Integrative medicine. I. Smith, Ava.
R733 .F86 2022
615.5--dc23

TABLE OF CONTENTS

PREFACE

This book has been written, keeping in view that students want more practical information. Thus, my aim has been to make it as comprehensive as possible for the readers. I would like to extend my thanks to my family and co-workers for their knowledge, support and encouragement all along.

The medical treatments which are used instead of traditional therapies fall under the umbrella of alternative medicine. This includes a wide range of health care products and therapies such as acupuncture, chiropractic, magnetic field therapy, etc. The diagnostic and therapeutic disciplines which are used in conjunction with conventional medicine are known as complementary medicine. Complementary and alternative medicine often use natural substances such as foods, herbs, animal and fungal products, minerals, nonvitamin supplements, and megavitamins. Some of the other medical practices which are classified as complementary or alternative are aromatherapy, Ayurveda, herbalism, diet therapy, naturopathy, homeopathy and yoga. The topics included in this book on complementary and alternative medicine are of utmost significance and bound to provide incredible insights to readers. It discusses the fundamentals as well as modern approaches of these fields. This textbook is a complete source of knowledge on the present status of these fields.

A brief description of the chapters is provided below for further understanding:

Chapter - Introduction

Alternative medicine is a form of medicine other than standard medicine which aims at achieving the healing effects of medicine. This is an introductory chapter which will briefly introduce alternative and complementary medicine as well as their benefits, usage, disadvantages and advantages.

Chapter - Traditional Medicine

The health practices, approaches, knowledge and beliefs which have been developed over generations for treatment, diagnosis and prevention of diseases are termed as traditional medicine. It incorporates plant, animal and mineral based medicines. The different types of traditional medicine such as traditional Chinese medicine, traditional Korean medicine and Iranian traditional medicine have been carefully analyzed in this chapter.

Chapter - Ayurveda

Ayurveda is a type of alternative medicine which was developed in the Indian subcontinent. It has eight major branches namely kaaya chikitsa, baala chikitsa, graha chikitsa, urdhaanga chikitsa, shalyaroga chikitsa, damstra chikitsa, jara tantra and vajikarana. The topics elaborated in this chapter will help in gaining a better perspective about these branches of Ayurveda.

Chapter - Naturopathy

Naturopathy refers to a form of alternative medicine which aims at creating a healthy and drugless system of healing based on various medical philosophies. It is used for treating diseases such as asthma and obesity. This chapter discusses in detail the treatment of these diseases through naturopathy.

Chapter - Homeopathy

Homeopathy is a medical practice that is based on the belief that the body can cure itself. It uses small amounts of natural products like plants and minerals to stimulate the healing process. Homeopathic dilutions and arsenic album are a few treatment derivatives used for healing. The topics elaborated in this chapter will help in gaining a better perspective about these aspects of homeopathy.

Chapter - Important Therapies in Alternative Medicine

There are various important therapies in alternative medicines such as acupressure, auriculotherapy, acupuncture, apitherapy, hypnotherapy, detoxification, ozone therapy, balneotherapy, halotherapy, etc. This chapter has been carefully written to provide an easy understanding of these therapies of alternative medicine.

Ava Smith

Introduction

CHAPTER 1

Alternative medicine is a form of medicine other than standard medicine which aims at achieving the healing effects of medicine. This is an introductory chapter which will briefly introduce alternative and complementary medicine as well as their benefits, usage, disadvantages and advantages.

ALTERNATIVE MEDICINE

Alternative medicine is a term that describes medical treatments that are used instead of traditional (mainstream) therapies. Some people also refer to it as "integrative," or "complementary" medicine.

Acupuncture

This is a traditional Chinese medicine technique that uses needles to stimulate specific points around the body. The person who performs this therapy (an acupuncturist) sticks thin, sterile needles into your skin. The goal is to help your body's natural healing process kick in. Studies show that acupuncture can be effective in treating a number of conditions, like neck and back pain, nausea, anxiety, depression, insomnia, infertility, and more.

Chiropractic Medicine

This practice focuses on the body's structure mainly the spine and how it functions. A trained professional called a chiropractor uses different techniques to adjust ("manipulate") your spine or other parts of your body so that they're in proper form, or alignment.

The goal of chiropractic medicine is to ease pain, improve body function, and help your body to heal itself naturally.

Much of the research around it has focused on low back pain. But studies show chiropractic can also be helpful for a number of other ailments, like headaches, neck pain, joint problems in your upper and lower body, and disorders caused by whiplash.

Energy Therapies

These focus on the energy fields many people believe exist in and around the body. Included in this category are:

Magnetic Field Therapy: This uses magnetic or electrical fields to treat a number of musculoskeletal problems. Studies show that it may work for osteoarthritis and other pain conditions. Some studies have even shown that it may help fractures heal faster. Magnetic field therapy may not be safe if you're pregnant, have an implanted cardiac device, use an insulin pump, or take a drug given by patch.

Those who practice this alternative treatment believe it taps into the body's natural energy to speed healing. The practitioner hovers his hands over your body or places them lightly on your skin. The goal is to channel energy through his hands to your body to promote healing. There's very little research to prove it works.

Herbal Medicine

This alternative therapy uses parts of a plant its roots, leaves, berries, or flowers - to heal the body.

According to the World Health Organization, an estimated 80% of people around the world use herbal medicine. Studies show certain herbs are effective in treating a number of health issues, like allergies, premenstrual syndrome, chronic fatigue, and more.

Unfortunately, herbal supplements can be sold without being proven to be safe or effective. Talk to your doctor if you're thinking about using them.

Ayurvedic Medicine

Ayurveda is one of the world's oldest medical systems. It started in India more than 3,000 years ago and is still widely used in that country today.

Those who use it rely on herbs, special diets, and unique practices to treat illnesses. But Ayurvedic products can also be dangerous. Researchers have found toxic minerals or metals, like lead, in some of the products.

There hasn't been enough research or clinical trials to support that Ayurveda works.

COMPLEMENTARY MEDICINE

Complementary medicine is the term used here to describe additional forms of treatment that may be given along with chemotherapy and traditional Western medicine.

Complementary medicine has claimed various types of "miracle" cures for cancer, which have since proved ineffective or even fraudulent. The integration of conventional and complementary medicine therapies however, is of increasing interest. This approach is being adopted at leading cancer treatment centers.

Sensory Complementary Medicine

Sensory complementary medicine therapies are therapies that work in conjunction with the five senses: smell, site, taste, sound and touch, as well as the body's overall energy.

Aromatherapy: The theory of this complementary medicine therapy is that the essential oils are absorbed into the body either through the pores of the skin during massage, or by inhalation through the nose. The scents released by the oil act on the hypothalamus, a part of the brain that influences the hormonal system. Thus, in theory, a smell might affect mood, metabolism, stress levels, and libido. Clinical research into claims for the effects of essential oils on medical conditions is not extensive, but the psychological effects of smell have been studied more.

Some common essential oils used are chamomile, lavender, peppermint, rosemary, sandalwood and tea tree. There are conflicting reports regarding the properties and uses for oils, and responses to smells are highly personal.

Landscape Therapy is the showing of peaceful, relaxing landscapes to patients, scenes that evoke calm and tranquility. They may be shown in a darkened room via a slide show or video screen, or they may be shown in the form of art books or actual artwork. Landscape therapy is often used as a distraction technique to help manage pain and anxiety.

Music Therapy is an expressive art form designed to help individual move into harmony and balance. Music therapy can incorporate both listening to and/or playing music. Music therapists are professionals who are educated to design music programs for patients. Through the use of music, individuals explore emotional, spiritual and behavioral issues. Music therapy can help patients release emotions and relax. Listening to music can be either calming or invigorating.

Massage is a form of complementary medicine that relies on the body's nerve endings and pressure points to promote relaxation. There are many forms of massage: Shiatsu, Hellerwork, and Reflexology for example. However, the most widespread variation builds upon the five basic strokes of Swedish massage: effleurage (slow, rhythmic gliding strokes in the direction of blood flow towards the heart) petrissage (kneading, pressing and rolling muscle groups) friction (steady pressure or tight circular movements, often used around joints) percussion, (drumming hands on body) and vibration (rapid movement shaking the muscle back and forth).

There are many benefits to massage therapy for patients undergoing treatment for cancer. There are also concerns and possible risks. Massage therapy has been used to treat stress and anxiety, improve mood, induce relaxation, and control pain. For patients undergoing surgery the application of appropriate massage can promote healing at incision sites and may prevent or reduce scarring. Use of foot massage was shown to have a positive effect on patients' perceptions of pain, nausea and relaxation.

There are situations in which massage can be risky or the techniques need to be adjusted. For example; massage should not be given if signs of infection are present at the surgical site. Immediately after surgery when a person is at risk of developing blood clots, massage of the legs is not advised. Patients undergoing radiation should not have massage techniques applied in the area of the radiation field because the massage may further irritate the irradiated skin. During chemotherapy, often patients are at increased risk of infection, anemia or bruising. Special precautions need to be taken with massage at this time. The use of massage therapy as an adjunct to cancer treatment should be discussed with the patient's treating physician (oncologist, radiation oncologist or surgeon). This is so that any risks can be discussed about the patient's condition can be provided so that a licensed massage therapist (LMT) can provide a safe and effective massage to the patient with cancer.

Therapeutic Touch is a complementary medicine form that presupposes that people have individual "energy fields" that interact with one another and with the environment as part of a universal energy force. These fields are thought of in scientific, rather than in mystical terms. In the late 1960's Dr. Dolores Krieger, Professor of Nursing at New York University learned the technique of "laying on of hands" from a healer, Dora Kunz. She began to teach what she called Therapeutic Touch to her students.

In a Therapeutic Touch (TT) session, the practitioner attempts to attune their energy fields with the patient so that disturbances in the "energy flow" are balanced and the body's healing powers can work freely. Hands are placed inches above the body and gently moved over it to assess any changes or blockages in the energy field. Using sweeping movements, the practitioner will try to treat the area of imbalance, perhaps by visualizing healing energy directed from her body to the patient. A session may last 10-15 minutes. TT is used to treat stress-related conditions, such as fatigue and headaches. It is also used for pain relief, especially from muscle strain and following surgery. It also has been used to promote wound healing, and for lymphatic and circulation disorders.

Reiki is a form of Japanese spiritual healing. This complementary medicine has its foundation in ancient Tibetan Buddhism, apparently forgotten until its rediscovery in the late 19th century. The aim of reiki is to promote health, maintain well-being, and help people attain a higher consciousness. Practitioners draw on "reiki energy" channeling it to areas of need in themselves and their patients. They borrow terminology from physics, claiming that reiki acts at an atomic level, causing the body's molecules to vibrate with higher intensity and thus dissolving energy blockages that lead to disharmony and disease.

A treatment session lasts about an hour; the practitioner directs reike energy through his hands to the patient. The patient lies clothed on a treatment table and the practitioner holds his hands on or over the body in 12 basic positions for about five minutes each. This is said to balance the body's energy centers or "chakras." Some patients may feel relaxed after treatment; others feel invigorated.

Reflexology: According to practitioners, the feet are a mirror of the body, and applying pressure to areas on the foot that correspond to the affected organs may help to relieve symptoms such as pain, constipation, and nausea. Reflexology is increasingly available in many hospices, and is often given by nurses.

Cognitive Complementary Medicine

Cognitive Therapy promotes mind-body healing by using the power of positive thinking to facilitate recovery. Types of cognitive therapy include:

Guided Imagery (visualization) is a process where the patient is assisted in imagining positive images and desired outcomes to specific situations. The practitioner works with the patient initially to discover what is they are trying to accomplish with the therapy. Then a mental image is created. For example, patients are asked to focus on feeling stronger or better, or to picture the destruction of tumor cells while in a state of relaxation. In one technique, patients visualize various aspects of treatment, from the least frightening to the most painful, remaining calm and relaxed at each step. This method has helped patients to control nausea before chemotherapy.

Hypnotherapy would be similar to guided imagery, however a physician or licensed hypnotherapist would be needed to induce deep relaxation.

Meditation is a method of relaxing and quieting the mind to relieve muscle tension and facilitate inner peace. There are numerous forms of meditation, taught individually or in group settings.

Relaxation and Deep Breathing: Patients are taught these types of complementary medicine techniques to help to release muscle tension, relieve breathlessness, lessen anxiety and encourage a greater sense of control, particularly when receiving unpleasant or stressful treatments.

Biofeedback: A training technique in which people are taught to improve their health and performance by using signals from their own bodies, is particularly found to be useful for managing pain and side effects.

Expressive Complementary Medicine

Expressive Therapies are treatments in which patients are encouraged to express their thoughts. Expressive therapies are thought to alleviate anxiety by allowing the patient to release fear and frustration in a positive, creative fashion. These therapies include:

Journal Writing: Writing in a journal is an effective way to handle some of the emotions that living with cancer triggers. Often people facing a serious illness find it difficult to express their feelings to others. Journal writing can allow a person to express difficult feelings in a safe and private way. Regular journal writing also helps people to clarify their thoughts and make good choices.

Art Therapy: Drawing, painting and sculpting, especially when carried out in a group environment, encourage pleasure in creativity and enable people to find a way of expressing their feelings that cannot be easily put into words.

Physical Complementary Medicine

Physical Exercise: When possible for the patient, physical exercise has been shown to release endorphins (mood elevating hormones) and promote better general health, relief of tension and positive attitudes. Even something as simple as walking and certain forms of dance have been helpful to patients.

Yoga is a form of gentle exercise consisting of body postures and breathing techniques. It has been practiced for thousands of years in India, and has now become popular around the world. In the West it is valued more for its physical than spiritual benefits, such as its ability to increase suppleness and vitality, and to relieve stress and fatigue.

T'ai Chi is a noncombative martial art that uses breathing techniques and sequences of slow, graceful movements to improve the flow of qi, or "life energy," calm the mind, and to promote self-healing. It is often described as "meditation in motion." It is practiced more as a form of preventive health care than as a response to an ailment.

Qi Gong is an ancient system of movement, breathing techniques, and meditation, which is designed to develop and improve the circulation of "qi" or "life energy" around the body.

Medical Systems Complementary Medicine

Medical Systems is an overall term used to describe the types of different, alternative, or non-traditional medicines that may be called upon in addition to western medicine. Some of these include naturopathy, Anthroposophical medicine, Western herbalism, Chinese herbalism, and ayurveda.

BENEFITS, USAGE AND DISADVANTAGES

Benefits and usage of Alternative Medicine

The natural therapies present in alternative medicines are age-old as compared to western form of treatments such as antibiotics and surgeries. According to physicians, most alternative medicine therapies started with clinical impressions or scientific research. The medicines are safe and involve natural substances. One primary objective of alternative medicines is to relieve people from depending largely on drug usage and help them manage their lives naturally. For users' convenience, below given are some ways to use alternative medicines:

1. People following an alternative medicine may do physical exercises such as osteopathy, yoga, infuse physical activity, tai chi, meditation and reflexology. To do these exercises, place the pillow on a surface providing comfort to the body, since these exercises stimulate and manipulate structural balance of the body. In addition, the exercises improve overall bodily functions. Users may practice these exercises for mental, physical, spiritual and emotional benefits.

2. Users may undergo massage therapy, which involves manipulating and rubbing the body tissue for mental and physical relaxation. They may do this either at home or at a massage clinic. When at home, apply massage oils to the neck, forehead, feet and hands.

3. Change the way of thinking. Exercise the mind first, so the body follows it. Meditate for relaxing the mind, thinking positively and clearing stress. Take deep breaths for better healing. Simultaneously, make use of enhanced visualization of objects for forming good thought patterns.

4. For relaxing the body, drink herbal teas. Improvement of bodily functions depends on what people eat and drink, since the same relieves, stimulates and has a healing effect on the body. Consume fresh fruits, vegetables and vitamins daily so that the body gets essential nutrients. Drink ginger tea since it is effective in the cure of nausea and heals the body naturally.

5. Those who wish to develop strong bones and healthy muscles may seek the help of a chiropractor. Chiropractic is a method of treatment that manipulates the body structures, especially the spine to relieve low back pain or even headache or high blood pressure. The chiropractor shows people their pressure points.

6. A simple, yet curable method that comes under alternative therapy is laughter as being the best medicine. People have experienced miraculous changes in certain health disorders due to mere laughing. As such, it is advisable people watch comedy shows on TV. Read magazines and books that promote laughter. Alternately, cleanse the entire body with essential oils, herbs, fruits that have certain therapeutic benefits on the skin. Combine herbs, natural products and fruits together as a remedy to skin disorders.

7. Users may try alternative medicines such as the electromagnetic therapy and biofeedback, which controls body functions such as heart rate, brain activity and blood pressure.

People have turned to using alternative medicine, since it offers multiple health benefits and cures them from long-term ailments in a natural way.

Disadvantages of Complementary Therapies

They Take Time to Work.

Most alternative treatments do not heal instantly. It usually takes several hours or even months before you can see any positive effects. This can be discouraging for some, especially if you have a nagging headache that you want to go away immediately. This is why some practitioners will not recommend complementary therapy for emergency situations.

They Require Lifestyle Changes

You have to commit your time, energy, and sometimes even your finances if you really want to adopt holistic medicine as your method for gaining optimum health. This means having to make some major changes to your lifestyle, such as changing your diet and adopting a different mindset when it comes to dealing with the stressors in life. But if this leads you to improved overall well-being, then maybe this can be more of an advantage than a disadvantage.

They might Interact with Certain Medication

Some herbal remedies might interact with prescription drugs, while some types of natural therapies might have contraindications for your existing condition. That is why you must always inform your conventional or complementary practitioner about the medicines you are currently taking and the true status of your condition, and ask for their professional advice regarding incorporating alternative therapies for your healing.

More conventional medical practitioners are becoming more open to the use of complementary therapies as supportive treatments. However, you must still make sure that you make informed decisions before adopting any form of treatment, whether it is conventional or alternative.

References

- What-is-alternative-medicine, guide, balance: webmd.com, Retrieved 31 March, 2019
- Complementary-medicine: chemocare.com, Retrieved 14 July, 2019
- Benefits-uses, alternative, medical: disabled-world.com, Retrieved 17 May, 2019
- 6-advantages-and-disadvantages-of-complementary-therapies: connectusfund.org, Retrieved 19 April, 2019

Traditional Medicine

CHAPTER 2

The health practices, approaches, knowledge and beliefs which have been developed over generations for treatment, diagnosis and prevention of diseases are termed as traditional medicine. It incorporates plant, animal and mineral based medicines. The different types of traditional medicine such as traditional Chinese medicine, traditional Korean medicine and Iranian traditional medicine have been carefully analyzed in this chapter.

Traditional medicine refers to health practices, approaches, knowledge and beliefs incorporating plant, animal and mineral based medicines, spiritual therapies, manual techniques and exercises, applied singularly or in combination, to treat, diagnose and prevent illnesses or maintain well-being. In the last decade traditional medicine has become very popular partly due to the long unsustainable economic situation in the country. The high cost of drugs and increase in drug resistance to common diseases like malaria, bacteria infections and other sexually transmitted diseases has caused the therapeutic approach to alternative traditional medicine as an option for concerted search for new chemical entities (NCE).

TRADITIONAL CHINESE MEDICINE

Traditional Chinese medicine (TCM) is a system of medicine at least 23 centuries old that aims to prevent or heal disease by maintaining or restoring yinyang balance. China has one of the world's oldest medical systems. Acupuncture and Chinese herbal remedies date back at least 2,200 years, although the earliest known written record of Chinese medicine is the Huangdi neijing (The Yellow Emperor's Inner Classic) from the 3rd century BCE. That opus provided the theoretical concepts for TCM that remain the basis of its practice today. In essence, traditional Chinese healers seek to restore a dynamic balance between two complementary forces, yin (passive) and yang (active), which pervade the human body as they do the universe as a whole. According to TCM, a person is healthy when harmony exists between these two forces; illness, on the other hand, results from a breakdown in the equilibrium of yin and yang.

A visit to a traditional Chinese pharmacy is like a visit to a small natural history museum. The hundreds of cabinet drawers, glass cases, and jars in a typical pharmacy hold an enormous variety of desiccated plant and animal material. In 1578 Li Shizhen published his famous Bencao gangmu (Compendium of Materia Medica), which lists 1,892 drugs and some 11,000 formal prescriptions for specific ailments.

The Practice of Traditional Medicine

To restore harmony, the Chinese healer may use any of a staggeringly large array of traditional remedies. The patient may be treated with acupuncture or acupressure, moxibustion (moxa treatment), or cupping (in which hot glass cups are placed on the patient to draw blood to the skin). The Chinese healer may prescribe a brew prepared with one (or some combination) of thousands of medicinal plants or dried animal parts (e.g., snakes, scorpions, insects, deer antlers) in the Chinese pharmaceutical armamentarium.

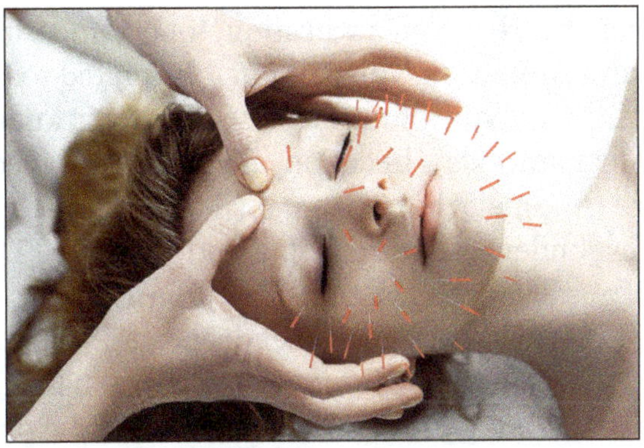

Acupuncture consists of the insertion of one or several small metal needles into the skin and underlying tissues at precise points on the body.

The Role of Qi and Meridians

An essential aspect of TCM is an understanding of the body's qi (life force; literally, "vital breath"), which flows through invisible meridians (channels) of the body. This energy network connects organs, tissues, veins, nerves, cells, atoms, and consciousness itself. Generally speaking, there are 12 major meridians, each of which connects to one of the 12 major organs in TCM theory. Meridians are also related to a variety of phenomena, including circadian rhythms, seasons, and planetary movements, to create additional invisible networks.

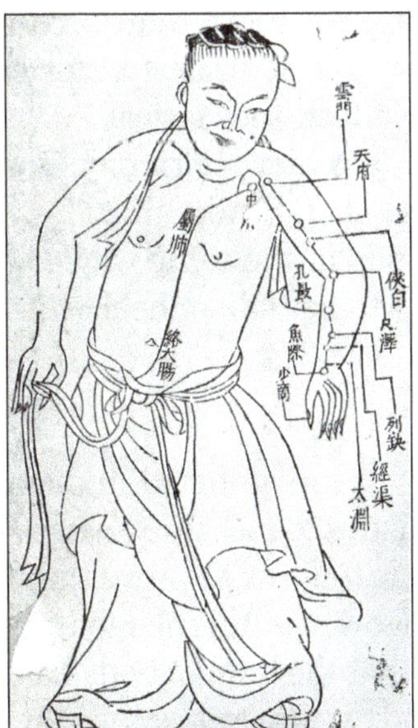

Acupuncture points.

In acupuncture thin needles are inserted into specific points along the meridians. The needles stimulate the meridians and readjust the flow of qi to balance the body's yin and yang. In place of needles, massage (acupressure) can also be used to stimulate the acupuncture points. Acupuncture is sometimes accompanied by moxibustion, the burning of small cones of an herb (typically Artemisia moxa) at acupuncture points. Not only can the meridian network be used to alleviate symptoms; it can also endow TCM with the ability to change consciousness in those who receive treatment.

A TCM practitioner uses smell, hearing, voice vibration, touch, and pulse diagnosis to discover the source of an unbalanced health condition, which organ it is related to, and which meridians are affected. In addition, the practitioner typically makes use of what is known as the five agents, or five phases (wuxing). By observing natural law in action, ancient healers recognized five basic elements in the world wood (mu), fire (huo), earth (tu), metal (jin), and water (shui) and found that these elements have myriad correspondences, both visible and invisible. This framework helps skilled TCM practitioners to identify unbalanced relationships. For instance, one key correspondence relates to time of day. If an individual always gets a headache at 4 PM, this signals that Bladder qi is unbalanced, since the Bladder (of the TCM Kidney/Bladder organ pair) is in charge of maintaining the body's functions at that time. Using the five-element theory, the practitioner can create a healing plan that might contain such components as acupuncture, herbs, lifestyle changes, and foods for healing. It might also include Chinese psychology, which shows how the energy of unbalanced emotions can affect proper organ function.

Herbal Therapy

TCM makes use of herbs and herbal formulas to strengthen organ function and support good health. An understanding of the essence of various herbal components gives the TCM practitioner a way to create a healing effect that reaches beyond the chemical composition and physical properties of the herbs. The practitioner chooses the herbal formula whose essence, or signature energy vibration, correctly stimulates or adjusts the body's own energy vibration.

Chinese herbal formulas, some in use for more than 2,200 years, are composed of ingredients chosen to function in combination with each other. In Western medicine, medications are usually prescribed individually for a specific effect. In classical TCM herbal formulas, each herb has a different purpose or role to help the body achieve harmony. For a plant to have been included in the Chinese apothecary, each of its parts had to be identified for a different healing purpose. TCM also looks at the healing properties of foods in the same way. Different foods carry different energies that can go directly to specific organs to help them heal.

Modern Developments

Various Western scientific disciplines have conducted studies to learn how Chinese medicine works, but it is difficult to use a Western yardstick to measure Eastern medicine. For example, many studies on acupuncture involve research that attempts to prove that this modality can eliminate or reduce pain or alleviate certain conditions. However, this elementary approach ignores the deeper insight and experience of Chinese medicine that the human body has unlimited healing power and that the complementary energies of health and disease reflect the yinyang principle within the human body.

Genetics Research and Drug Development

The yinyang principle can be applied to a genetic disease such as inherited breast cancer and its associated genes BRCA1 and BRCA2. According to this principle of natural law, if either of these genes is activated, somewhere in another part of the genetic code there also exists a gene to fix the action of the cancer gene, because there is an opposite energy to the one that produced the disease. There must be complementary programs running one for developing the disease and one for healing it.

Nearly 200 modern medicines have been developed either directly or indirectly from the 7,300 species of plants used as medicines in China. For example, ephedrine, an alkaloid used in treating asthma, was first isolated from the Chinese herb mahuang. Today, scientists continue to identify compounds in Chinese herbal remedies that may be useful in the development of new therapeutic agents applicable in Western medicine. For example, an alkaloid called huperzine A was isolated from the moss Huperzia serrata, which is widely used in China to make the herbal medicine qian ceng ta. Studies suggest that this agent may compare favourably with manufactured anticholinesterase drugs such as donepezil, which are used to treat Alzheimer disease.

Meditation and Health

The meditation exercises tai chi (taijiquan) and qigong ("discipline of the vital breath") are examples of other integral features of traditional Chinese healing that have been incorporated into health and fitness programs to complement modern medicine. Tai chi is characterized by deliberately slow, continuous, circular, well-balanced, and rhythmic movements that were originally practiced as a martial art. Qigong, which was known in ancient China as "the method to repel illness and prolong life," contains elements of meditation, relaxation training, martial-arts techniques, and breathing exercises that are intended to cultivate qi and transmit it to all the bodily organs. Today, many people worldwide regularly perform these exercises to promote health and may indeed derive health benefits from the exercise and relaxation.

TRADITIONAL KOREAN MEDICINE

Traditional Korean medicine refers to the traditional medicine practices that originated and developed in Korea.

Korean medicine traditions originated in ancient and prehistoric times and can be traced back as far as 3000 B.C. when stone and bone needles were found in North Hamgyong Province, in present-day North Korea. In Gojoseon, where the founding myth of Korea is recorded, there is a story of a tiger and a bear who wanted to reincarnate in human form and who ate wormwood and garlic. In Jewang Ungi, which was written around the time of Samguk Yusa, wormwood and garlic are described as 'edible medicine', showing that, even in times when incantatory medicine was the mainstream, medicinal herbs were given as curatives in Korea. Medicinal herbs at this time were used as remedial treatment such as easing the pain or tending injury, along with knowing what foods were good for health. Moreover, wormwood and garlic are not found in ancient Chinese herbology, showing that traditional Korean medicine developed unique practices and inherited them from other cultures.

In the period of the Three Kingdoms, traditional Korean medicine was influenced by other traditional medicines such as ancient Chinese medicine. In the Goryeo dynasty, a more intense investigation of domestic herbs took place: The result was the publication of numerous books on domestic herbs. Medical theories at this time were based on the medicine of Song dynasty, but prescriptions were based on the medicine of the Unified Silla period such as the medical text First Aid Prescriptions Using Native Ingredients or Hyangyak Gugeupbang, which was published in 1236. Other medical journals were published during this period like Introductory Guide to Medicine for the General Public or Jejungiphyobang.

Medicine flourished in the period of the Joseon. For example, the first training system of nurses was instituted under King Taejong, while under the reign of King Sejong the Great measures were adopted to promote the development of a variety of Korean medicinal ingredients. These efforts were systematized and published in the Hyangyak Jipseongbang, which was completed and included 703 Korean native medicines, providing an impetus to break away from dependence on Chinese medicine. The medical encyclopaedia named *Classified Collection of Medical Prescriptions*, which included many classics from traditional chinese medicine, written by Kim Ye-mong and other Korean official doctors from 1443 to 1445, was regarded as one of the greatest medical texts of the 15th century. It included more than 50,000 prescriptions and incorporated 153 different Korean and Chinese texts, including the *Concise Prescriptions of Royal Doctors* which was written by Choi Chong-jun in 1226. *Classified Collection of Medical Prescriptions* has very important research value, because it keeps the contents of many ancient Korean and Chinese medical books that had been lost for a long time.

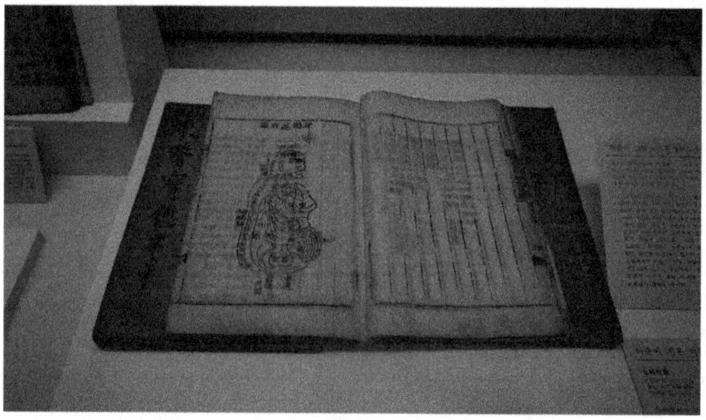

Dongui Bogam, National Museum.

After this, many books on medical specialties were published. There are three physicians from the Joseon Dynasty who are generally credited with further development of traditional Korean medicine Heo Jun, Saam, and Lee Je-ma. After the Japanese invasion in 1592, *Dongeui Bogam* was written by Heo Jun, the first of the major physicians. This work further integrated the Korean and Chinese medicine of its time and was influential to Chinese, Japanese and Vietnamese medicine.

The next major influence to traditional Korean medicine is related to Sasang typology. Lee Je-ma and his book, *The Principal of Life Preservation in Oriental Medicine* systematically theorized with the influence of Korean Confucianism and his clinical experiences in Korea. Lee Je-ma said that even if patients suffer the same illness, patients need to use different herbal applications to treat the same illness due to the pathophysiologies of individuals. He stresses that the health of human body had a close relationship with the state of mind. He believed that the human mind and body were not separate and they closely reflected each other, and the aspect of mind needed to be considered when examining the causes of disease. Thus, not only food and natural environment but also emotional changes in humans can be another major reason for illness. He believed that medical diagnosis and treatment should be based on person's typology rather than on symptoms alone and each person should be given different prescriptions depending on the constitution of the individual. Sasang typology focuses on the individual patients based on different reactions to disease and herbs. Treat illness by the treatment of the root cause through proper diagnosis. Key to this diagnosis is to first determine the internal organs or pathophysiology of each patient.

The next recognized individual is Saam, a priest-physician who is believed to have lived during the 16th century. Although there is much unknown about Saam, including his real name and date of birth, it is recorded that he studied under the famous monk Samyang. He developed a system of acupuncture that employs the five element theory.

In the late Joseon dynasty, positivism was widespread. Clinical evidence was used more commonly as the basis for studying disease and developing cures. Scholars who had turned away from politics devoted themselves to treating diseases and, in consequence, new schools of traditional medicine were established. Simple books on medicine for the common people were published.

Lee Je-ma classified human beings into four main types, based on the emotion that dominated their personality and developed treatments for each type:

- Tae-Yang or "greater yang"
- So-Yang or "lesser yang"
- Tae-Eum or "greater yeum"
- So-Eum or "lesser yeum"

Methods

Herbal Medicine

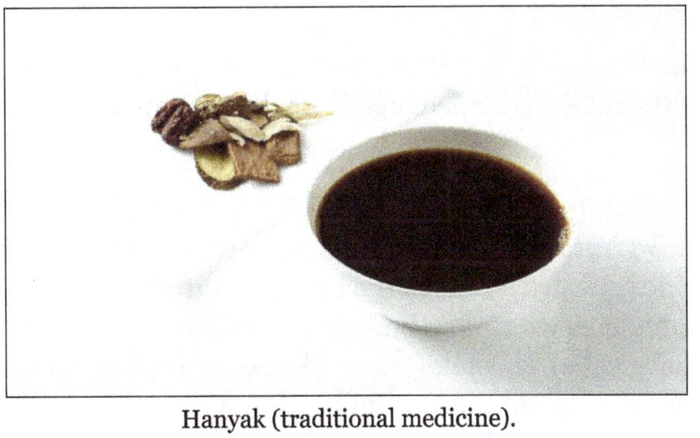

Hanyak (traditional medicine).

Herbalism is the study and practice of using plant material for the purpose of food, medicine, or health. They may be flowers, plants, shrubs, trees, moss, lichen, fern, algae, seaweed or fungus. The plant may be used in its entirety or with only specific parts. In each culture or medical system there are different types of herbal practitioners: professional and lay herbalists, plant gatherers, and medicine makers.

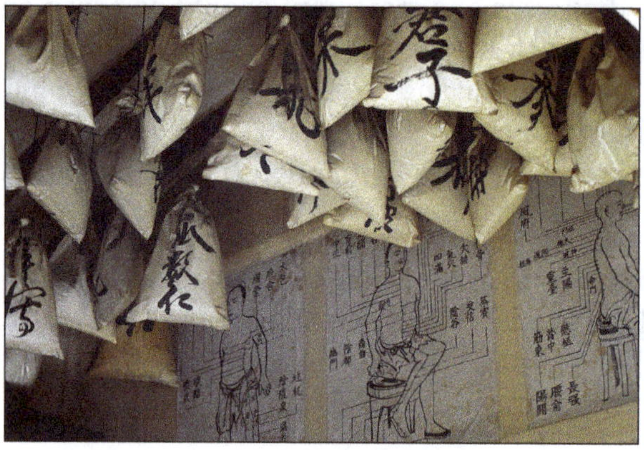

Doctor's office in folk village.

Herbal medicines may be presented in many forms including fresh, dried, whole, or chopped. Herbs may be prepared as infusions when an herb is soaked in a liquid or decocted simmered in water over low heat for a certain period. Some examples of infusion are chamomile or peppermint, using flowers, leaves and powdered herbs. Decocting examples may be rose hips, cinnamon bark, and licorice root consisting of fruits, seeds, barks, and roots. Fresh and dried herbs can be tinctured where herbs are kept in alcohol or contained in a vinegar extract. They can be preserved as syrups such as glycerites in vegetable glycerin or put in honey known as miels. Powdered and freeze dried herbs can be found in bulk, tablets, troches similar to a lozenge, pastes, and capsules.

Non-oral herbal uses consist of creams, baths, oils, ointments, gels, distilled waters, washes, poultices, compresses, snuffs, steams, inhaled smoke and aromatics volatile oils.

Many herbalists consider the patient's direct involvement to be critical. These methods are delivered differently depending on the herbal traditions of each area. Nature is not necessarily safe; special attention should be used when grading quality, deciding a dosage, realizing possible effects, and any interactions with herbal medications.

An example of herbal medicine is the use of medicinal mushrooms as a food and as a tea. A notable mushroom used in traditional Korean medicine is Phellinus linteus known as Song-gen.

Acupuncture

Acupuncture is used to withdraw blood or stimulate certain points on humans and animals by inserting them on specific pressure points of the body. Traditional acupuncture involves the belief that a "life force" (*qi*) circulates within the body in lines called meridians. Scientific investigation has not found any histological or physiological evidence for traditional Chinese concepts such as *qi*, meridians, and acupuncture points, and many modern practitioners no longer support the existence of life force energy (*qi*) flowing through meridians, which was a major part of early belief systems. Pressure points can be stimulated through a mixture of methods ranging from the insertion and withdrawal of very small needles to the use of heat, known as moxibustion. Pressure points can also be stimulated by laser, massage, and electrical means.

Moxibustion

Moxibustion is a technique in which heat is applied to the body with a stick or a cone of burning mugwort. The tool is placed over the affected area without burning the skin. The cone or stick can also be placed over a pressure point to stimulate and strengthen the blood.

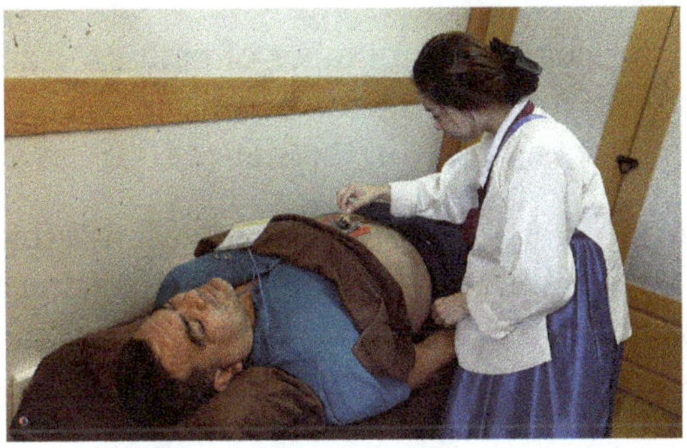

World Traditional Medicine Expo.

A Cochrane Review found limited evidence for the use of moxibustion in correcting breech presentation of babies, and called for more experimental trials. Moxibustion has also been studied for the treatment of pain, cancer, stroke, ulcerative colitis, constipation, and hypertension. Systematic reviews have found that these studies are of low quality and positive findings could be due to publication bias.

IRANIAN TRADITIONAL MEDICINE

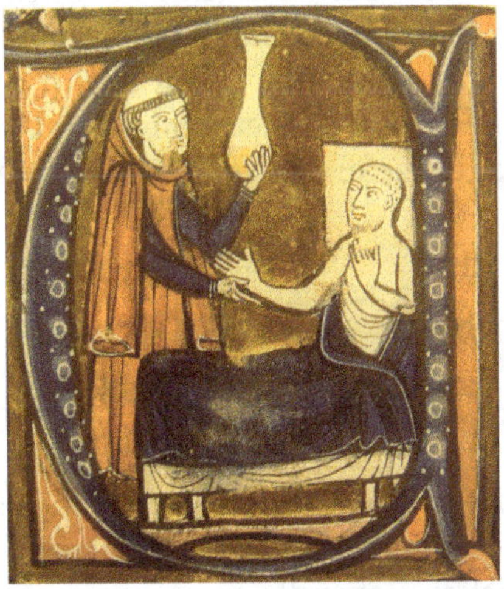

Rhazes browsing urine samples of patients.

Iranian traditional medicine (ITM), also known as Persian traditional medicine, Iranian-Islamic traditional medicine (IITM), traditional Iranian medicine (TIM), or simply traditional medicine is one of the most famous and most ancient forms of traditional medicines. Studies and research reveal that some of the earliest records of history of ancient Iranian medicine can be found from 8,000 to 6,500 B.C., while Hippocrates, a physician considered one of the outstanding figures in the history of medicine, dates to about 460 BC.

Iranian traditional medicine is grounded in the four humours concept: Phlegm (Balgham), Blood (Dam), Yellow bile (Ṣafrā') and Black bile (Saudā'). Some traditional medicine forms are in this base. Yunani and Graeco-Arabic are the most famous of that. It is based on the teachings of physician Hippocrates and Roman physician Galen, and developed by Rhazes, Avicenna (Ibn Sena) into an elaborate medical system.

The old medical system was developed by a number of nations. Iranian traditional medicine, although often presumed as part of unani medicine because of a great overlap between these two, still is a separate tradition with roots further in the ancient Iranian and Indian past.

Kiarash Aramesh of Edinboro University of Pennsylvania, states that efforts for revitalizing TIM in recent years have shaped two main attitudes: academic medicine and quakery, the latter advocated by figures such as Hossein Ravazadeh. While many academics use evidence-based scientific measurements, there is also psuedoscientific stream in the academia.

Principles

As it is religiously obligatory to know the rudimentary rules and regulations set by Islam, it is also mandatory for all human beings to familiarize themselves with basics regarding healthcare to avoid illnesses as much as possible, and treat mild illnesses to prevent refractory and chronic disease.

The lifestyle rules in Iranian traditional medicine are mainly focused on six core principles or six most essential items also known as Setah Zaroriah in Persian. Food and drinks, climatic conditions and environment, physical activities and rest, Iranian traditional medicine, psychiatric conditions including those of sadness, happiness, depression, stress, sleep and wakefulness, absorbing key nutrients and ridding body from waste materials (through sweat, urine, or feces) are the six fundamental and guiding principles behind the Iranian traditional medicine lifestyle, and issues one must take into account while trying to maintain their health. The first step to ensure optimum health is recognizing one's temperament (physical and mental characteristics from Iranian traditional medicine point of view) to get useful information to find the best route to a healthy life.

Temperament

Mizaj (Temperament)

Iranian traditional medicine is a holistic medicine which has been based on individual differences, a determinant basic concept named as mizaj (temperament), a set of physical and mental characteristics defined by examining one's symptoms and signs in the past and in the present. According to Iranian traditional medicine everybody has a definite mizaj which is determinant to construct all physical or mental characteristics. Generally, mizaj represents the excess or lack of warmness and humidity in one's body and is classified into four categories - also called four qualities - of warmness, coldness, dryness and wetness. Mizaj is a spectrum, meaning that two persons might have warm mizaj but one's mizaj might be warmer than the other one. In fact, no two individuals have exactly the same mizaj, however they can resemble one another to some extent. Relatively speaking, mizaj and genetics are similar in that once an embryo starts to develop, its mizaj will be determined. Consistently the parents' mizaj can also be a deciding factor in the child's mizaj which is also referred to as the "inherent" or "main" mizaj with which one is born.

While mizaj is forming, one or two of the four qualities of warmness, coldness, dryness, and wetness might become dominant and decide the main mizaj. Therefore, regarding which quality is more dominant, the tempers are classified into nine categories of warm, cold, wet, dry, warm and dry, warm and wet, cold and dry, cold and wet, and moderate (when none of the qualities are dominant).

There are no absolute good or bad temperaments, and as long as they are within their normal range - reflected in physical and mental health - they are in a balanced (normal or good) state. So, each individual should maintain their own balanced state during their life by choosing the kind of lifestyle which suits them best by corresponding to their own distinguishing mizaj. As each person's mizaj differs from another one's, people's lifestyles will necessarily be different; this is the main essence of the Iranian traditional medicine in maintaining health and treating illnesses.

By adopting the kind of lifestyle which fit each person's mizaj one should try to keep the inherent warmness and humidity of their body in certain range (as per their main mizaj) and avoid possible "mal-temperament" (or s'ou-e-mizaj).

Mizaj is not just confined to human beings but literally every object, situation, and state in the world has a defining mizaj which has an impact on human beings' health.

Determining Temperament

The tempers (amzajeh) are classified into nine categories: moderate, warm, cold, wet, dry, warm and dry, warm and wet, cold and dry, cold and wet.

Displaying some identifying behavioral and physical characteristics would describe one's temperament.

Frame

- Being stout, sturdy, big-boned and prone to gain weight are signs of wetness, while not gaining weight and being thin are the distinguishing characteristics of dryness.

Body Parts

- Bigger faces, fingers, lips, noses, organs, and body parts are defining characteristics of people with wet mizaj whereas people with dry mizaj have smaller body parts.

Complexion

- A rosy and ruddy complexion is a sign of warmness and wetness, while having a yellow cast is sign of warmness and dryness; on the other hand, a light and fair complexion is a distinctive characteristic of people with wet and cold mizaj. People with a dark complexion have a cold and dry mizaj.

Hair

- People with dry mizaj have coarse, curly and coily hair; warmness causes the hair to grow faster and people with warm mizaj have thick black hair, with thick density and more volume. Silky, straight, smooth, thin and fair hair which grows slower is a distinctive characteristic of people with cold mizaj. Wetness would cause the hair to easily hold a curl or style.

Skin

- People with dry mizaj have dry skin, and people with wet mizaj have soft and squishy skin. Having naturally high body temperature once someone touches people with warm mizaj tells they are warm. People with cold mizaj feel cold and run colder than other people and once someone touches them can tell they are colder than normal.

Activity

- Warmness brings about an increase in exuberance and energy levels, which boost speech and body movement and speed, while coldness causes quite the reverse symptoms, as people with cold mizaj don't have much energy and are generally slow, and take their time speaking and acting.

Mental Traits

- People with warm mizaj are normally and usually more extroverted, sociable, and less patient, while people with cold mizaj are more introverted, calmer, and more patient. People with warm mizaj are more inclined to suffer stress and restlessness; however, people with cold mizaj have a tendency to experience depression and melancholic thoughts and may have hallucinations or sometimes delusions.
- However, keep in mind that one's personality traits may be modified or changed due to various factors such as upbringing, religion, spirituality, and one's striving to change their attitude. Therefore, one's personality may not necessarily match their temperament.

Sensitivity

- People with warm mizaj are more sensitive to warmness (surrounding environment, foods and drinks); those with cold mizaj are more sensitive to coldness; those who have dry mizaj are more sensitive to dryness and those with wet mizaj are more sensitive to humidity.

Sleep

- Sleeping too much or sleepiness is a sign of wetness and needing much less sleeping hours is a defining characteristic of dryness.

Waste Matter

- Waste matters (e.g. urine, sweat, and feces) in those with warm mizaj have strong color and odor while in people with cold mizaj the waste matters don't have strong color or odor.

Everything has a Temperament

Organs's Temperament

All organs and body tissues have a specific Mizaj.

- Heart: The heart has a warm and dry temperament. The constant movement of the heart throughout one's life is a proof of its warmness. Consuming too much of food stuff with warm Mizaj such as pepper and spices would give the person palpitations. Having a fixed shape and being stiff and firm are the signs of the heart dryness.

- Brain: The brain, command center for the human nervous system, is cold and wet. The brain is composed of water in addition to the squashy and soft gray and white matter. The brain is capable of transmitting great deal of signals without failing. The way the brain is operating and its shape all are defining its cold and wet Mizaj. Consuming too much dairy products such as yoghurt, water, and fruits and vegetables with high water content such as water melon, peach, or lettuce would increase coldness and humidity in the brain and result in sleepiness and impair its performance.
- Blood, liver, muscles: These organs are warm and wet. They are pretty warm and flexible and in order to protect them, stay healthy, and keep on living one must consume meat, bread and fairly sweat food items which all have warm and wet Mizaj. However, overeating and consuming too much of the aforementioned food items would cause a build-up of waste materials in these organs which would manifest themselves by displaying symptoms of polycythemia, fatty liver disease, muscle stiffness and inflammation in muscles.
- Bones, teeth, fingernails, and hair: They all have cold and dry Mizaj. They are firm and rigid and in order to protect and reinforce them and build strong bones and teeth one must consume food stuff with cold and dry Mizaj such as essential minerals (magnesium, calcium, zinc, iron, etc). Such minerals are normally found in Kashk (dairy product made from drained yogurt), wheat and rice bran, almond, and barley. Therefore, due to their Mizaj, these organs are sensitive to coldness and dryness. Coldness and dryness could bring about pain in bones in cold weather, toothache by having something cold, and brittle and dry hair and nails.

Colors Temperament

Colors have temperament, meaning that they can reveal the real temperament of the objects or intensify the temperament of the individuals.

The color yellow is the symbol of warm and dry temperament and red represents warm and wet Mizaj. On the other hand, dark colors such as black, grey, and brown symbolize cold and dry Mizaj and bright colors such as white and blue are the symbols of cold and wet Mizaj.

Warm colors (red, orange, and yellow) are signs of warmness and can increase the temperature in a confined area. These colors are associated with danger, threat, warning, and movement and the way they affect the brain they increase metabolism and heat in the body and put it on alert which from Iranian traditional medicine point of view are sign of excessive heat.

Therefore, those with cold Mizaj who normally have slow metabolism, and feel sluggish had better use warm color for their clothes and houses while for people with warm Mizaj the reverse is true. People with warm temperament who are normally vibrant, brisk, lively and stressed should avoid using such colors and use cool colors such as white, blue, and light green. Such cool hues can bring about a more passive reaction in the brain and can make a person feel pleased and relaxed. Accordingly, cool colors do not suit people with cold temperament.

Seasons Temperament

Each season has a defining temperament and that's why they differ from one another dramatically. So individuals must take special measures depending on the seasons.

- Spring: Spring is warm and wet. Individuals, especially those with warm and wet Mizaj, should avoid consuming sweets, fatty, greasy, and heavy food stuff and food items with warm Mizaj during spring. Instead they had better to eat light food with cold Mizaj.
- Summer: Summer is warm and dry. Abstaining from food stuff with warm Mizaj and sun exposure, and using food stuff with cooling characteristics and taking enough rest particularly for people with warm and dry Mizaj is highly recommended during summer.
- Autumn and winter: Autumn is cold and dry and winter is cold and wet. Those with cold Mizaj should take better care of themselves during these seasons. Cutting back on food stuff with cold Mizaj such as sour foods, dairy products and citrus fruits and staying away from cold places is recommended to people with cold Mizaj. On the other hand, consuming sweets and food stuff with warming characteristics such as spices, getting exercise and staying in warm places is of benefits to them.

Day and Night Hours

The amount of warmness and humidity fluctuate over days and nights, therefore different temperaments form: morning is cold and wet, before noon is warm and wet, afternoon is warm and dry and evening and night are cold and dry. The various Mizaj of the day and night are the reasons behind mood swings and pain or discomfort varying during the day and night.

Flavors

Flavors have temperaments and accordingly would cause warmness, coldness, dryness and wetness in the body. One can simply decide the Mizaj of a food item or a drink by tasting them to a great extent.

Tasteless food items, also called watery, are cold and wet. Every insipid food item such as lettuce, dairy products such as yoghurt, or doogh (a yogurt-based beverage) and citrus fruits which are not too much sour or sweet are cold and wet.

Sour flavor is cold and dry and cause dryness and coldness in the body as well. Vinegar and pickled vegetables and fruits preserved in vinegar, sour fruits or sour juices, verjuice, and Qarehqurut or black kashk (fabricated from the liquid yoghurt) are all cold and dry.

Salty, bitter and spicy flavors which are usually used to give foods a special taste are warm and dry. Although spicy foods are warmer and dryer than bitter and salty foods respectively.

Sweet flavor is warm and wet and most food items (including main dishes and high-calorie food) are classified in this group and that's why many people like sweet food and drinks.

With that being said people with cold and dry Mizaj (melancholic temperament) who are normally thin and don't gain much weight with dark complexion and rough and dry skin, particularly in autumn (a cold and dry season) and in mountainous areas should avoid consuming sour foods and drinks or they are most likely to develop conditions such as dry skin, depression, and weakness.

Same goes for people with other temperament, for instance, people with warm and wet Mizaj (sanguine temperament) should cut back on sweet food stuff, people with warm and dry Mizaj (choleric temperament) should avoid using much spices and salt, and people with cold and wet Mizaj (phlegmatic temperament) must use dairy products, water and citrus fruits cautiously.

Climates

Each climate has its own unique temperament. In general polar regions, mountainous areas with rocky landscapes and sandy grounds and north winds are cold and dry. Salt marshes and deserts are warm and dry. Coastal areas are cold and wet and the tropics are warm and wet.

In Iran, southern, some eastern and mostly central areas which are getting the most sunlight and low humidity are warm and dry. Coastal areas in southern Iran and northern Iran (only during hot seasons) are warm and wet. Western and northwestern areas which are dominantly mountainous are cold and dry and coastal areas in northern Iran (except for warm seasons) are cold and wet.

The house orientation, whether the house is south-facing or north-facing or built underground determines the house temperament. North-facing houses (in Iran) with less sun exposure, underground houses or houses built in damp and humid places are cold and wet or cold and dry. But south-facing houses which get enough sunlight and built in warm places are normally warm and dry.

Even winds can develop a distinguishing temperament in an area. Winds blowing from northern and north western areas in Iran are cool and can cause a cold temperament while winds blowing from southern areas are warm and develop a warm and wet temperament in a place. Western and eastern winds are moderate and won't change the temperament much so it's better for the windows to be on the west and east sides of the house in Iran to get the eastern and western winds.

The type of soil of an area also counts. Areas with loamy and clay soil which have great potential of retaining water are wet while areas with chalky or sandy soil composed of the large particles which prevent it from retaining water are warm and dry.

Psychiatric Conditions

Any changes in the psychiatric condition affect human's temperament to some extent. The longer and deeper the conditions are the more dramatic and lasting the effects are. On the other hand, changes in one's temperament would influence psychiatric condition as well.

By releasing the heat from inside the body to the surface and vice versa and by absorbing heat from the body's surface such psychiatric conditions would cause warmness or coldness in the body.

Anger and excitement increase warmness and dryness in the body and are the signs and also the cause of dry and warm Mizaj as someone with warm and dry Mizaj is more prone to get angry or excited. People who consume too much warm and dry food stuff might be affected by anger and excitement more often.

Therefore, all lifestyle tips for warm and dry Mizaj (temperament) would apply to anger and excitement as two psychiatric conditions. Eating spicy, sweat, salty, deep fried and roasted food stuff especially in warm seasons would trigger anger and excitement.

Pleasure and worry are warm and wet while fear, horror, and depression can be a result or sign of cold and dry or in some cases cold and wet Mizaj.

Someone who is suffering from depression tends to sleep to evade the sad thoughts and this would cause wetness in the body. People who are preoccupied, cynical, pessimistic, skeptic, or experience mental or emotional instability must know that they might either have a cold temperament or consume too much food stuff with cold and wet or cold and dry Mizaj.

These people should cut back on dairy products, watery and sour fruits and other food stuff of the kind. Instead they had better use food and hot drinks with warm temperament. Kebabs, spices, salty and spicy food, cinnamon tea, saffron tea, mint tea, or ginger tea suits such people as the fear and the sadness they feel caused by cold Mizaj of their brain or body would go away and they feel more courageous and fearless.

One should not necessarily experience the fear or anger, even imagining such psychiatric conditions would produce the same result.

In order to maintain mental health one can both practice self-control and seek professional help and consultations. But more importantly adopting a lifestyle that suits one's Mizaj by consuming foods and drinks in accordance with their temperament is very important in keeping mental health.

If someone with warm Mizaj keeps eating food stuff with warming characteristics particularly during warm seasons it is not very unlikely for them to lose their temper. So in order to remain healthy, both physically and mentally, one should firstly reconsider and reform his or her lifestyle and diet and then seek professional help or study more deeply about the situation.

Exercise, Lack of Movement

Moderate exercise would increase the heart rate and breathing (respiratory) rate, excrete sweat from the sweat glands which then evaporates off of the skin, more blood is able to near the surface of the skin making the skin feel warm and look red and finally make people often feel so at ease and cheerful. All these are symptoms of warm temperament which means taking exercise would lead to warmness in the body.

But high-intensity exercise would drive the body to excessive coldness, weakness, getting blue face or lips after exercise; moreover after heavy exercise heart rate would take much longer to return to base which is not healthy.

Additionally, as getting exercise would increase heat in the body the humidity and other unwanted materials would excrete from the body through the bowels or the skin which result in dryness so taking exercise would do much good to people with warm and wet Mizaj (sanguine temperament) who are stout, sturdy, and burly with muscular body and also cold and wet Mizaj (phlegmatic temperament) who have coldness and wetness in their bodies. Although in general getting them is of benefit to everyone.

On the contrary, lack of movement slow the metabolism and humidity and waste materials would accumulate in the body and drive the temperament to coldness and wetness which is accompanied by weakness, lethargy, obesity, and puffiness.

Certainly compared to light and mental exercises such as swimming and chess, vigorous and outdoor exercises such as football, and running have warmer and drier temperament.

In general, from Iranian traditional medicine point of view, anaerobic exercises which consist of short exertion and high-intensity movement would mostly increase the heat in the body and won't decrease the wetness much so they best suit people with cold Mizaj and don't help much in losing weight. On the other hand, exercises which are of light-to-moderate intensity and can be performed for extended periods of time would decrease the wetness and increase the heat in the body and therefore those with warm Mizaj who want to lose weight would benefit such exercise.

Sleeping and Wakefulness

Sleep is a passive, dormant part of our daily lives while wakefulness is daily recurring brain state and state of consciousness. Sleep is physical and mental rest and wakefulness is the state of physical and mental activity.

Therefore, the longer one stays up the drier and warmer their bodies get and the longer one sleeps the wetter the brain and the body gets and their temperament would drop lower. Actually while one is sleeping the body temperature drops meaning that the heat would move from the surface of the body and that's why one might need a blanket during night. During the day the heat would move to the surface of the body and the body temperature raise.

In any cases that one is forced to get less sleep (having to study for an exam, being under mental pressure or having to finish a project) the brain and the body would get warmer and drier so in order to control the excessive warmness or dryness in the body one should cut back on warm and dry food stuff. Additionally taking a short nap during the day (20 minutes) especially in warm climates and seasons is highly recommended to them.

Besides, those with cold and wet Mizaj should not sleep much as long sleep would increase wetness in the body. People with phlegmatic temperament should cut down on food items cold and wet temperament to sleep shorter and get up easily and not having trouble waking up. They had better wake up once or twice during the night so that wetness would not build up in their bodies.

Age Range

Although each person is born with a fixed and unique temperament, also called inherent or main Mizaj, with the passage of time the main Mizaj is subjected to fluctuation. For example, someone's Mizaj might get drier but this doesn't mean that they are suffering mal-temperament.

Taking that into account, in addition to the main Mizaj, one must take heed of the temperament of the age as well and take necessary actions to stay healthy.

Growth Period

- Based on Iranian traditional medicine since one is born until the age 25 to 30 is called the "growth period" with the preponderance of warmness and wetness. To keep teenagers and children healthy they are recommended to consume food stuff with warm and wet Mizaj. Eating bread, meat, rice with bran, fruits especially apple and sometimes banana is good for them. However, one should be careful to avoid excessive warmness.

- As one is growing up in this period they need to consume more food and increase their nutrient intake. Eating diverse types of foodstuffs and high quality food is of importance to this age group.

Youth

- From age 30 to 40 is called "youth" when the wetness will dwindle and the warmness and dryness will be more dominant. One should not use much food stuff with warm and dry Mizaj as it increases the yellow bile in the body.
- Many might break out in pimples, get irritable, and suffer sleep deprivation. Such people should abstain from spices, pepper, spicy food stuff, sweets, salty and deep fried food items. Instead they should use food stuff with cooling characteristics such as pomegranate, pomegranate juice, sour cherry, peach, lemon, lime juice, barberry juice, verjuice, lettuce, sekanjabin (Iranian drink made of honey, mint and vinegar), vegetable soups and dairy products such as yoghurt to moderate the warmness and dryness in the body. They can also use lifestyle tips for people with choleric temperament.
- During growth period and youth one has a strong digestive system and can easily digest heavy food such as meat.

Middle Age and Old Age

- Between the age 40 to 60, called "middle age", warmness and wetness will plummet and instead, coldness and dryness will be predominant in the body. After the age 60, also called "old age", abnormal wetness may occur in the body so the *Mizaj* will become cold and wet. And due to the excessive wetness for many old age is synonymous with puffy eyes and face, loose skin, drowsiness and loss of memory.
- In some other cases coldness and dryness will be more predominant in the body. Therefore, the coldness and dryness affiliated with the old age would cause wrinkles, curvature of the spine, drop in body temperature, poor digestive system, and puffy eyes and face.
- Generally with the old age, comes decrease in warmness and wetness and the temperament of people aging over 60 will get colder and drier compared to their main Mizaj. That's why lifestyle tips for people with melancholic or phlegmatic temperament would also suit people age over 60.
- Due to their poor digestive system the elderly should abstain from fatty food, leftovers, deep fried foods, fast foods, tomato paste and sauces, and conserves and instead they should consume high calories and low volume foods. They should also cut back on water, dairy products, fruits with cooling characteristics, and sour food items.
- They had better eat vegetables, celery, chives, fig, grape, raisin, walnut with fresh cheese, and almond porridge with honey or rock candy, fresh bread, lamb meat, meat extract,

almond, pistachio, coconut and coconut extract, fruits such as sweet apple, grape, partridge and quail meat.

- Eating Abgoosht (Iranian stew made with lamb, chickpeas, white beans, onion, potatoes, and tomatoes, and dried lime) provided that it is not too fatty and is cooked well with cumin and apple is recommended to the elderly. Eating wheat Haleem (a stew made of wheat and meat) and drinking goat warm milk with honey also suit them. However, they should avoid drinking cold milk while they are hungry.
- In order to avoid constipation which is pretty normal at old age, eating plum or fig which are soaked together and drinking sweet almond oil or olive oil is of benefits.
- Applying moderate oils such as sweet almond oil or violet oil (for people with warm inherent Mizaj) on the body surface is also good for these people. Wet cupping therapy is not recommended to these people unless a physician order in a special condition.
- People over 40 must know that they had better follow lifestyle tips for old age and take them more seriously after age 60.

Mal-temperament

Spoiling one's inherent or main Mizaj and moving towards excessive warmness, coldness, wetness or dryness, would undermine the persons' health. So one must take immediate action by recognizing the factors causing such symptoms and prevent them from developing.

In case one fails to keep his/her Mizaj within its normal range for a long time, mal-temperament or 'So-e-Mizaj' will strike the body and diseases will progress.

Excessive Warmness

There are cases when the patient is diagnosed with excessive warmness in their bodies. Here are reasons as to why someone might experience conditions caused by excessive warmness in their bodies:

- Heavy and fast exercise, intense activity, and getting too much high speed massage.
- Great anger or happiness.
- Being exposed to heat, either sun, or fire for a long time.
- Consuming food stuff with warming characteristics or warm Mizaj such as date, pepper, etc.
- Clogged pores which reduce sweat.
- Infection and infectious diseases which cause fever and excessive body heat.
- Having a warm temperament, as people with warm Mizaj are more prone to be affected by warm Mizaj food stuff or warm environment than people with cold Mizaj.

Fast heart rate, breaking out in pimple and mouth ulcers, and sleep deprivation are the side effects of excessive warmness.

Excessive Coldness

Some actions or consuming some food stuff can contribute to excessive coldness in the body:

- Lack of movement or not taking exercise.
- Profound sadness and disturbing thoughts which lead to sleep deprivation and restlessness.
- Intense mental or physical activity which will first increase the warmness but will ultimately result in nutrient deficiency and lack of warmness in the body.
- Being in cold, dark and damp places.
- Eating, and drinking food stuff with cold Mizaj or rubbing cold ointments for long time.
- Taking too many showers or baths which unclogs the pores, work up a sweat, and decrease the warmness in body.
- Not eating much or going on starvation diet.
- Overeating which slows digestion and decrease warmness in the stomach; poor digestive system would not efficiently convert food to energy, bad materials build up in body and the body would become cold.

Unfortunately people with cold Mizaj can soon be affected by mal-temperament caused by excessive coldness by consuming food stuff with cold Mizaj.

Excessive Dryness

Below is the list of reasons one might suffer conditions sparked by excessive dryness:

- Factors contributing to increased warmness, such as being adjacent to fire, intense activities and heavy exercise which raise the warmness and correspondingly deplete the body of its natural humidity.
- Being stressed out, overexcited, and feeling ecstasy as well as being preoccupied and sleep deprived.
- Dry climate and seasons such as summer and autumn and residing in dry areas such as mountains and deserts.
- Construction jobs and pottery and being in close contact with soil, stone and building materials.
- Being in close contact with paint and solvents especially painters and those working in labs.
- Consuming food stuff with dry Mizaj such as vinegar or salt, or applying volatile substances such as oil, gasoline, alcohol, ether, acetone, hair color and nail polish topically.
- Not eating much (fasting for long time) as the body is unable to gain and maintain normal level of humidity.

It is worth mentioning that thin people with dry and cold and dry and warm Mizaj are more likely to suffer from excessive dryness.

Excessive Wetness

On the other hand, some actions and eating some foods and drinks can lead to excessive wetness in the body.

- Lack of movement and not taking exercise which would cause excessive wetness built up in the body, getting swollen and puffy and not being able to rid of it.
- Staying long in wet places such as bath or swimming pool.
- Wet climate or seasons such as spring and winter or residing in coastal areas.
- Being in close contact with water, for instance by working in paddy fields, teaching swimming, or being a lifeguard.
- Consuming too much food and drinks with wet Mizaj such water, dairy products, vinegar, sour food, lettuce, peach, and nectarine as well as rubbing oils with wet Mizaj such as violet oil.
- Overeating as the digestive system is not capable of converting the food into energy properly and that unwanted materials and humidity will build up in the body.
- Decrease in the amount of body waste (sweat, menstrual fluid, urine, feces) discharged from the body which causes excessive wetness in the body.

Again, overweight people with wet Mizaj are more prone to suffer excessive wetness.

Choleric, Sanguine, Melancholic and Phlegmatic

In the Iranian-Islamic traditional medicine the excess or less of warmness and humidity define four essential temperaments of "Warm and Wet (sanguine or Damawiy)", "Warm and Dry (choleric or Safrawiy)", "Cold and Dry (melancholic or Saudawiy)" and "Cold and Wet (phlegmatic or Balghamiy)" respectively. The terms in the parentheses refer to four groups of material in the body (called "humors" or 'Akhlat') including blood, yellow bile, black bile, and phlegm respectively. Words written in italic show original Persian terms in the ancient literature.

Choleric: Warm and Dry

- People with choleric temperament are usually tall and thin. They have a small frame, for instance, their fingers, lips, and other body parts are not much big and they are unlikely to get overweight.
- They have a dry and warm skin color with yellow and sometimes peachy undertone.
- They have rapid pulse, are exuberant, quickly finish what they are supposed to do usually perfectly and carefully and speak fast.
- People with warm and dry Mizaj mostly feel hot and have naturally high body temperature.
- Due to the dryness of their Mizaj they might suffer constipation and waste matter (urine, sweat, and feces) discharged from their bodies usually has strong odor and color.

- Burning in the anus and urinary tract can be common among this group.
- Due to the warmness in their body they soon digest food and as they don't have adequate amount of nutrient supply to provide the energy needs of the body they soon get hungry and irritated if they don't get enough food timely.
- Normally their mouth gets dry soon.
- Due to the warmness in their body which moves upward to the head their hair grow faster. They have coarse thick black hair. Premature graying and hair loss is prevalent among these people.
- As they're able to think fast and act fast, they might lose concentration to some extent, in other words they may undertake multiple tasks at the same time and give up some of them halfway through them. Accordingly, they might be pegged as hyperactive.
- They have keen senses and can easily notice the smallest changes in smells, voices, taste, color, etc.
- They are overly sensitive and will be easily upset or offended by events or things that people say and must be treated delicately.
- They don't need much sleep and actually seem fine and ready for work with a little amount of sleep. They are not very sound sleepers and are prone to suffer stress, anxiety, and sleep deprivation.
- They are idealist and fond of efficiency. They are also in favor of punctuality as well. Once they make an appointment they are always worried not to get there on time.

Lifestyle Tips

- People with warm and dry Mizaj are better not to consume deep fried food stuff specifically during hot seasons.
- Choleric people should not consume large amounts of food stuff such as pepper, garlic, cinnamon, and ginger as well as spicy and salty foods. They are better not to eat much sweets either.
- They should also consume small amounts of red meat and abstain from eating other hot Mizaj meat with warming characteristics such as camel, quail and partridge meat as much as possible.
- Although honey is of great benefits, those with warm and dry Mizaj are not recommended to take too much of it particularly during hot seasons; however, eating honey in cold seasons is fine for them.
- Tomato paste and sauces, specifically hot and chilly sauces, are pretty harmful for such people. They should use egg (especially yolk) the least possible during summer.
- Considering their Mizaj eating Abdoogh Khiar (a cold cucumber and yogurt soup) is highly recommended for these people during summer. Of course eating too much of it might cause flatulence.

- Additionally, eating vegetables such as lettuce and other summer fruits with cooling characteristics (cold Mizaj) is recommended as well. However, they have to be cautious about eating vegetable with warming characteristics (warm Mizaj) such as tarragon, leek, cress which also have strong tastes.
- In general people with warm and dry Mizaj can experience a healthier life by consuming food stuff with cooling characteristics such as sour or sweet-and-sour food items and drinks like barberry juice, raspberry juice, or pomegranate juice, liquid chicory extract (Kasni) and fumitory extract (Shahtareh), as well as flixweed.
- Such people should avoid direct sun exposure; warm colors such as yellow and red either of their clothes or their surrounding environment would stimulate and increase their internal heat.
- Watching thrillers and rock music are not recommended to these people.
- Placing drops of violet, zucchini or coriander oil in each nostril or rubbing the oils on the face is of benefits for this groups.
- Taking daily showers proved to be advantageous for people with choleric temperament as the wetness of the shower would help to balance the warm and dry Mizaj of these people.
- Accordingly, floating in water for example in a cold tub, swimming pool, or bath tub as well as using cool moisture humidifiers could be of benefits for these people. However, it is ill-advised to use a dry sauna.
- Staying up for long hours, engaging in intense activities, and being stressed out and anxious which will all increase the heat in the body should be avoided as much as possible particularly in hot seasons and warm climate.

Sanguine: Warm and Wet

- People with sanguine temperament are normally gregarious, sociable and cheerful. They are usually in high spirits, beaming and funny, patient, and adaptable.
- They have rosy and ruddy complexion and soft and smooth skin. They also have thick black hair, with thick density and more volume which can easily hold a curl or style.
- People with sanguine temperament are stout, sturdy, and burly with muscular body.
- These people have bigger veins which are prominent and easily seen through the skin in the arms and legs. They also have a more powerful and stronger pulse.
- They rarely get sick; however, they are more prone to develop diseases such as obesity, hypertension, blood clots, high cholesterol, and high uric acid.
- Drowsiness, particularly in spring, is pretty common among people with sanguine temperament.
- They are more likely to get abscess or pimple.

- They are good leaders and due to their wetness, they are patient and very well manage and cope with those inferior or superior to them.
- Their bodies feel squishy and warm.
- Those with warm and wet temperament have good appetite and have a craving for meat, bread, rice and in general wider selection of dishes.
- Waste matter (urine, sweat, and feces) discharged from their bodies have usually strong color and odor. As they consume food in large quantities they expel more body waste.

Lifestyle Tips

- Similar to people with choleric temperament, those with sanguine temperament had better not consume large amounts of food with warming characteristics (warm Mizaj) especially in warm seasons and warm climate.
- Consuming high calorie and heavy food items, such as red meat, camel meat, turkey, large amounts of bread and rice and liver especially during spring and summer (warm days) is not recommended to this group.
- In general, diet high in starchy foods such as pasta, potato, and egg is not very much to the benefit of sanguine people. People with warm and wet Mizaj should consume butter, cream, sweats, salty and spicy foods the least.
- Different kinds of ash (a thick soup or stew, which is usually served hot) such as rice ash, verjuice ash, sumac ash, pomegranate ash, Sekanjabin (one of the oldest Iranian drinks; a syrup made of boiled water, sugar and vinegar) ash, soups, broths and stews, light vegetarian cooked or steamed food, and Abdoogh Khiar (a cold cucumber and yogurt soup) are best for them.
- Heavy ash such as ash-e Reshteh (a thick soup with thin noodles, vegetables and beans, cheakpea, lentil, etc.) or ash-e Shole Ghalamkar (another thick soup with beans, peas, lentils, leafy vegetables, rice, etc.) and Haleem (a stew which includes wheat or barley and meat as main ingredients) are not of much benefit for these people. Only light ash with small amounts of beans, fresh vegetables and slight sour taste are recommended to people with warm and wet Mizaj.
- Fasting and even in some cases skipping lunch (however cautiously) would be beneficial for these people. They should wait for hunger to hit them in order to eat.
- They should consciously avoid being in warm and humid conditions such as sauna, steam room, or a bathroom filled with steam.
- As they have muscular body and a body composition of larger proportion of muscle tissue rather than fat they need to exercise and lack of movement would cause waste products and other toxins to build up in their bodies. Therefore, they are more prone to develop high uric acid and cholesterol levels.
- Consuming low-calorie food stuff which only fills one up without gaining weight such as light stews, celery, carrot, olive, lettuce, cabbage, broccoli, spinach, and zucchini are recommended to this group of people.

- People with warm and wet Mizaj are advised to donate blood and receive wet cupping therapy. As a general rule, enhancing body's natural ability to detox through main exit routes for toxins such as urine, feces, and perspiration is pretty good for this group.
- Drinking liquid chicory extract (Kasni), fumitory extract (Shahtareh), sour and sour-sweat Sekanjabin, pomegranate, lemon, or barberry syrups would also benefit them.
- Vegetables, salads and watermelon are also good provided they don't over eat. Consuming sour fruits and adding sour food items to stews and ash would be of advantage to them.

Melancholic: Cold and Dry

- People with melancholic temperament are usually thin and have a small frame. They don't have much big body parts and they don't gain weight.
- They have a dark complexion and are likely to develop dark spots on their skin. Their skin is dry and rough and is prone to get wrinkles and show signs of premature skin aging.
- Their hair is coarse, curly and coily. They also have excessive unwanted hair (hirsutism).
- From mental point of view people with melancholic temperament tend to be introspective and introvert. They act and speak unhurriedly and might need more time to accomplish a task but they do it perfectly.
- They might have negative thoughts. They can be perceived as cynical, skeptic, distrustful and suspicious and are more likely to develop mental disorders such as depression. They are also likely to have more nightmares than other people.
- They don't sleep much, have trouble falling asleep fast, they have a lower sleep efficiency which might cause disturbed sleep. They have a retentive memory.
- They are much more likely to suffer constipation and dry skin. Body waste discharged from their bodies (including urine, feces, menstrual fluid or sweat) might become dark in color. They are not in favor of change. For example, they try to wear the same clothes and perfumes as much as possible.
- They are sensitive to food stuff and drinks with cold and dry temperament and they have to cut down on pickled fruits and vegetables, food stuff with vinegar content, lentil, eggplant, leftovers, and fast food.

Lifestyle Tips

Lifestyle tips fitting people with melancholic temperament are listed below.

- People with melancholic temperament should not stay in dark and dim places for long.
- They should not take cold showers and stand in front of an air cooler. Living in warm and humid areas suit these people.
- Watching thrillers, tragedies and horror movies and reading tragedies might have some adverse effects on them.

- They had better to spend their lives by visiting family and friends, going to picnics, watching comedies and wearing colorful clothes and in general have fun.
- Wet cupping therapy is not recommended to this group as they usually suffer mild anemia and weakness to some extent.
- They should abstain from fast food, vinegar, pickled food with vinegar content, eggplant, cabbage, and mushroom.
- Consuming meat with moderate Mizaj (not warm or cold) such as lamb, fresh wheat bread, sweat fruits, cardamom, cinnamon, and nuts especially pistachio and almond is advantageous to them.
- Taking regular but gentle and light exercise is of benefits for them, however exercising in a cold gym or under strong sun is not good for them.
- People with cold and dry temperament should not wear perfumes with cooling characteristics such as violet or lilac, but wearing rosewater perfume is agreeable to their temperament.
- To decorate their houses they can use colorful tableaus.

Phlegmatic: Cold and Wet

- People with phlegmatic temperament usually feel cold and run colder than other people.
- They are light, fair and smoothed-complexioned and relatively speaking they have fine, glowing, radiant, and flawless skin. They have silky, straight, smooth and thin hair. They don't have much unwanted hair.
- Their body parts are big. They are normally bulky and quickly gain weight with a body composition of larger proportion of fat rather than muscle tissue and they usually seem swollen. They take their time thinking, speaking and acting.
- They oversleep and as they get up they feel they haven't got enough sleep. They usually have trouble waking up and they wake up tired.
- These people are prone to wake up with swollen feet, hands and puffy face specially after sleeping in the evening.
- They feel dizzy and tired early morning particularly when it's cold or they have consumed food or drinks with wet Mizaj such as yoghurt, sour food stuff or Doogh (a savory yogurt-based beverage popular in Iran).
- They usually are more sensitive to cold and humid weather. They are sensitive to dairy products, sour foods, large amounts of water, and high-water-content foods and should cut back on them.
- Due to the wetness of their bodies and brains, they tend to have a poorer and shorter memory compared to people of other temperaments, as wetness and coldness would result in decrease in transferring and storing data.

- People with cold and wet Mizaj are endlessly patient and calm and can put up with people with all sorts of belief.
- They expel fairly large amount of waste matter (urine, sweat, and feces) but the waste matter don't have strong color or odor unless waste materials have built up in their bodies.
- They don't have much strong pulse, neither do they have prominent veins. They also tend to suffer low blood pressure.

Lifestyle Tips

- Eating food stuff with cold and wet Mizaj is not recommended to people with phlegmatic temperament especially during cold seasons and in cold climate.
- In general they had better not to consume watery food such as soup or ash (kind of Iranian soup featuring noodle, beans, and vegetables) and stews. They should also try not to eat too much pasta, potato, and rice which would cause them to gain weight.
- They should abstain from dairy products (cheese, yoghurt, or doogh - a savory yogurt-based beverage), sauces, mayonnaise, sour paste or sour food items.
- Eating vegetables or fruits with cold Mizaj such as watermelon, cucumber, peach, plum, lettuce, and spinach is of no benefits to them, however, eating sweat fruits such as banana, apple, and quince would be advantageous to them.
- Consuming low-volume high calorie food such as salted or roasted almond, pistachio, raisin, and fig is good for them. Taking food stuff such as fig, melon seeds, radish, and thyme that trigger diarrhea or urination which could lessen the wetness in their body and create a feeling of lightness and joy is recommended to this group.
- They should cut back on thick food such as barely soup, kalleh pacheh (a dish of boiled cow or sheep's feet and head) and tripe. Instead, eating high calorie and low-volume food such as Kabab Barg (a Persian style barbecued and marinated lamb dish), Kabab Chenjeh (pure meat and very similar to western steaks usually made from the meat of newly slaughtered sheep, when it's still soft and fresh) egg yolk, and quail.
- They had better have mint, chives, tarragon, or mountain vegetables such a thyme or other vegetables grow in local areas as well as onion and garlic with their meals which all have warm Mizaj, suit their temperament and help them fully and easily digest their food.
- Adding salt and spices such as pepper, cinnamon, saffron, and ginger into their food is also of benefits to them.
- Being in cold and humid places such as bathtub, swimming pool, cold tub, and steam sauna is not good for them, while taking intense exercise such as jogging, running, cycling especially under low sun is recommended to them.
- While sleeping they had better use a hard mattress, use blanket, cover their head or sleep near to a heater with their head closer to it.
- Sleeping uninterruptedly for long hours would increase wetness in the body so people with phlegmatic temperament had better to get up during the night and then go back to sleep again.

- Sleeping during the day especially in autumn and winter is not advised to these people. They should sleep in warmer places relatively stretching the body and soft sports after getting up is beneficial to them. Doing this in the morning would decreases the chances of dizziness, tiredness, puffiness, Post Nasal Discharge (PND) and memory loss.
- Wearing perfumes with warm and strong scents as well as wearing clothes with warm colors such as red, yellow and orange is advised to them.
- People with cold and wet Mizaj need warmness and blood (which is a very warm substance) in their bodies so they are ill-advised to undergo bloodletting therapies such as wet cupping therapy, phlebotomy and leech therapy. Cupping therapy without taking any blood is all right.
- Watching sad, horror and philosophical movies is not appropriate for these people while watching comedies and thrillers which increase the warmness in the body very well suit them.

Humors

Humors, or to use the Pesian term 'Akhlat', are liquid humors formed in the liver and gastrointestinal system following digestion. In other words, after eating and drinking, digestion, the process of breaking down food stuff into smaller units and converting them into a substance suitable for absorption, happens.

Afterwards the substances move towards the liver and will be processed again (called the second digestion in traditional medicine) which form the four liquid humors called: blood, yellow bile, black bile, and phlegm.

So the gastrointestinal tract, also known as digestive tract, plays an important role in one's health and that's why it is said that all diseases begin in the gut. The four aforesaid humors, or *Akhlat*, are supposed to supply the cells and the body organs with necessary nutrients.

Therefore, the healthier the humors are the healthier the body. So, selecting healthy food stuff in accordance with the main Mizaj (temperament) to aid digestion is the point to keep healthy. Excessive amounts of blood, yellow bile, black bile, and phlegm is rooted from the fact that someone has not stick to their healthy diet.

In the Iranian traditional medicine 'abstaining' is the best path to effective treatment. According to a saying by Imam Reza, the eighth Shia Imam, once you are aware of the detrimental effects of a food item you should abstain from it and it is wise "not to choose your desire over your body's comfort".

Akhlat have Mizaj

As mentioned previously everything around us in this world has Mizaj and Akhlat are no exception. Akhlat can be also examined according to their warmness and humidity :

- Yellow bile is warm and dry, in case it increases in the body the body will become warmer and drier.
- Blood is warm and wet, excessive blood will surge warmness and humidity in the body.

- Black bile is cold and dry, similarly with copious amounts of black bile the body will get drier and colder.
- Phlegm is cold and wet, high amounts of phlegm in the body will rise coldness and humidity in the body.

Yellow Bile

- Yellow bile is not as abundant as phlegm and blood in the body. It is the lightest of all humors. It resembles cooking foam. Yellow bile acts as a diluent and facilitates the transfer of blood and nutrients from capillaries to the remote body organs.
- It is also in charge of metabolism of fats and lipids and ease digestion. Yellow bile is tasked with cleaning up the digestive system, vascular tissues, and genitalia. That's why people with excessive yellow bile might experience burning sensation with urination or defecation, frequent urination, frequent bowel movements, and heavy or prolonged menstrual bleeding.
- Thick or viscous blood cannot effectively flow into the small vessels and capillaries and provide the tissues with sufficient oxygen and nutrients, so it could cause lack of energy (fatigue) along with bruising or discoloration, cold feet, and cold hands. Yellow bile would stop such health conditions by improving blood circulation as its job is to accelerate the transfer of blood and nutrients in the body. Being hot and dry, yellow bile is accompanied with movement and motion rather than immobility.

Excessive Yellow Bile Symptoms

- Before describing the symptoms that might appear owing to the excessive yellow bile in the body it is worth mentioning that by having one of the symptoms one might not necessarily suffer excessive yellow bile but it doesn't mean that one must display all the symptoms at the same time to be diagnosed with excessive yellow bile either. Experiencing one or some of the symptoms might be the reasons for excessive black bile.
- On the other hand, one might suffer excessive yellow bile along with other humors namely blood, black bile or phlegm and report symptoms which may occur due to the various humors excess that stem from today's unhealthy lifestyle. Therefore, one might exhibit symptoms for excess of one or more humors.
- Another point is that one might suffer some of the symptoms which seems to be relating to excess of humors but they might be actually experiencing another condition.

Here are the symptoms that develop by excess of yellow bile in the body:

- Yellowing of the skin and eyes; feeling bitter taste in mouth; getting acne on the face or the scalp; having dry skin, eyes, mouth, nasal passages and bad breath; getting wrinkles; dark circles under the eyes; losing appetite; feeling nauseated, itching, burning, and irritation in genitalia or rectum; getting thin; feeling unquenchable thirst; troubled sleep; sleep deprivation; feeling stressed out; pins-and-needles sensation in fingers and/or toes and strong smelling waste materials (urine, sweat, menstrual blood) are some of the symptoms which appear by excessive yellow bile.

What to Eat what not to Eat

- Food stuff with warming characteristics (warm Mizaj), spicy food, overly sweet or greasy food, foods that are easy to digest such as well-baked wheat bread and young birds' meat specially in warm and dry season of summer can constitute to formation of fairly large amounts of yellow bile in the body.
- Those who are affected with excessive yellow bile should abstain from food stuff with warming or drying characteristics namely, spices, pepper, ginger, spicy vegetables such as garlic, onion, tarragon, and green cress, too much salt, sautéed or deep fried food, nuts such as walnut, hazelnut and peanut, sweet food stuff such as honey, red meat such as lamb, chicken, quail, partridge, or camel meat.
- On the other hand, consuming sour food stuff such as sekanjabin (an Iranian traditional syrup made of honey or sugar and vinegar), verjuice, sour or sour-sweet tamarind, lettuce, cucumber, zucchini, spinach, coriander, sour fruits and fruits with high water content such as citrus fruit, greengage, black mulberry, sour apple, blackberry, sour cherry, tangerine, sour orange, water melon, white meat and food with barely or mung bean would benefit this group of people.
- Generally adapting the lifestyle suitable for people with choleric temperament would suit people with excessive yellow bile.

Blood

"Blood" is the most abundant and accordingly the most important humor in the body which will be formed by eating main dishes. The humor of "Blood" is necessary for growth especially in children and teenager when growth spurt happens. So they will be needing larger amounts of "Blood" by consuming food stuff which will produce this humor in the body.

A great deal of the bloodstream is made up of humor of "Blood" which is warm and wet. It is noteworthy that the body lives on "Blood" as it keeps the body warm and moist as warmth and humidity are indicatives of being alive.

Excessive "Blood" Symptoms

- Similar to any other humor excessive amounts of "Blood" will cause discomfort or even serious illnesses. Dizziness, lightheadedness, frequent yawning, fatigue, red and bloodshot eyes, redness of the face and lips, blood filled pimples, abscess especially on the hips, genitalia or anus, bleeding of the gums while brushing your teeth, frequent nosebleeds, high blood pressure, losing mental acuity, a sweet taste in the mouth specially in the morning, heavier than normal or prolonged menstrual bleeding, itching, and hot and moist skin are of the symptoms of excessive "Blood".

What to Eat what not to Eat

- Consuming food stuff in accordance with one's Mizaj (temperament) would enable them to remain healthy.

- Though we might eat various food stuff the stable food which constitute to main dishes lead to the formation of "Blood" in the body. Wheat and wheat bread, rice, beans and chickpea, sweat fruits such as fig and grape, read meat specially lamb and beef, liver, kidney and heart meat, egg, fatty food stuff such as butter and cream, nuts like walnut and almond would produce "Blood" in the body. Consuming proportional amounts of such food items would normally produce "Blood" in the body and maintain the healthy state and growth.

How to Reach Baseline Level of "Blood"?

- As mentioned on multiple occasions Iranian traditional medicine highlights that abstaining and not consuming food and drinks which are not good for us depending on our main Mizaj are playing a major role in keeping healthy and in this case keeping baseline level of "Blood".
- Nowadays due to the lack of movement attributed to the modern life and consuming high amounts of food many suffer from excessive "Blood" and other Akhlat in their bodies and feel full all the time; in Iranian traditional medicine the feeling is called "Emtela" which means fullness in English.
- So, people especially those with warm and wet Mizaj (sanguine temperament), should not consume large amounts of food products with warm and wet Mizaj which produce excessive amounts of "Blood" in the body. Fasting and starving are of the treatments recommended to people suffering excessive "Blood". Therefore, decreasing food intake drastically for a fortnight would benefit them.
- Having a diet consisting of low calorie foods makes you feel full to help you ward off hunger. Food such as soups and stews with small amounts of rice, split peas, and fresh vegetables accompanied with natural laxative such as plum, tamarind, barberry juice, or sumac extract added half an hour before serving the food would help diminish excessive "Blood".
- Such food is called 'deceptive food' in Iranian traditional medicine as they deceive the one who eats them by making them think they are eating something but they don't actually gain any weight. They can be helpful in weight loss diets as well.
- Vegetable, zucchini, or okra stews which taste sour by adding verjuice, lemon, barberry, plum, tamarind, as well as salads and dairy products, drinking sour juices namely sour cherry and barberry, and homemade pickles provided they are not very spicy would benefit people experiencing excessive "Blood".
- Also wet cupping or bloodletting and donating blood prescribed or recommended by a skilled traditional medicine specialist proved to be effective in decreasing excessive "Blood" in the body.

Black Bile

- Black bile is cold and dry. It is sparse in the body but it sure is pretty essential for the body. The right amounts of black bile keep bones healthy and strong and that's why bones, teeth and tendons primarily live off black bile.

- Normal amounts of black bile also supports hair and nails, in fact black bile strengthen body parts, therefor, lack of black bile in the body will compromise bone's strength and the tendons function. In worst-case scenario it can lead to osteoporosis. Its shortage would also cause tooth decay and hair falling. Black bile also it stimulates appetite when the stomach is empty.

Excessive Black Bile Symptoms

- Darkening of the skin, developing brown skin patches, wrinkles, having dull skin, developing dark circles under your eyes, suffering muscle cramps (specially muscles of the posterior leg and toes during sleep), more painful menstrual cramps, irregular menstrual cycle, having depressing and negative thoughts, poor sleep, having nightmares, darker waste materials (sweat, urine), constipation, fake hunger, thicker and darker blood, having excessive unwanted hair, getting thinner, developing mental disorder such as depression, obsession, isolation, skepticism, and cynicism are symptoms of built up excessive or abnormal black bile in the body.

Black Bile Producing Foods

- All canned foodstuff, leftovers, fast foods containing sausages and deli meat (in general precooked and processed meats), frozen meat which are kept for a long time in the freezer, meet of old animals, salted or smoked fish can produce black bile in the body. Generally the older a food stuff is the more black bile and waste material it produces in the body and the harder it will be to digest.
- Fast foods, all kinds of sauces, and pickled fruits and vegetables are not good for people with excessive black bile and increase it in the body.
- Additionally, all kinds of sauces, food with additives, junk food such as chips, gumdrops, too much coffee, black and strong tea, vegetables such as eggplant, cabbage, cauliflower, tomato, green pea, corn, lentil, sour fruits, pickled vegetables and fruits, vinegar, too much cold water and ice, too much yogurt, sour doogh (a savory yogurt-based beverage popular in Iran), kashk (fabricated from the liquid yoghurt), and old sour cheese would result in production of black bile in the body.
- It is worth mentioning that black bile production in cold seasons, especially autumn, and cold climates such as mountainous regions normally increases.

How to Avoid and Treat Excessive Black Bile

- Clearly people suffering excessive black bile should avoid consuming food stuff which increase the aforesaid humor in the body.
- In case they are used to consume such food stuff they should try to modify their bad eating habits step by step in order to become healthy.
- People with melancholic temperament or those who suffer excessive black bile should eat foods with warm and wet temperament more and consider such food items in their food

choices. Abgoosht (Iranian stew made with lamb, chickpeas, white beans, onion, potatoes, and tomatoes, and dried lime), lamb kebab, quail, partridge, chicken or sheep heart (one should not consume too much liver or kidney because of their bad effects on the body tissues), soft-boiled or sometimes fried egg, wheat and wheat bread, haleem (a stew including wheat or barley and meat), ash (a traditional slow-cooked, thick soup made with chickpeas, beans, noodles, and fresh herbs), chick pea and beans and food containing them, sangak bread (bread made from whole-wheat flour) with some butter or animal fat or oil, sweet food stuff such as date or grape syrup, rock candy, homemade jams, sweet fruits, raisin, grape, quince, apple, melon, fresh fig, fresh or dried berries, vegetables such as basil and tarragon, nuts like almond, peanut, and hazelnut, almond porridge made with or without milk, spices used to give cardamom, cinnamon, and ginger would increase warmness and humidity in the body and help get rid of the built up black bile.

- Eating food stuff with warming characteristics which also increase the humidity in the body such as raisin, soft-boiled egg, and ginger can help people suffering excessive black bile.
- Eating natural laxatives such as olive oil or fig soaked in rosewater in order to rid the body of the waste material would also help ease excessive black bile symptoms. Rubbing sweet almond oil on the body especially in the shower or placing it in nostrils would greatly help treat dry skin and membranes. It would also ease the nerves and improve sleep quality.

Phlegm

- After the humor of blood, phlegm is the second most abundant humor in the body which has a cold and wet Mizaj.
- Phlegm is a slimy liquid very much like water (colorless, odorless and tasteless) and it can be found in body parts such as dermis, adipose tissue (body fat), synovial fluid, and the mucus lining the lungs, throat, mouth, nose, etc. which require humidity and flexibility to function properly.
- The cerebrospinal fluid which is the clear, colorless body fluid found in the brain and spinal cord is also made up of phlegm.
- One of the advantages of the phlegm is that by the temperature rise in each body part it can turn into the humor of blood and can feed that specific organ, so phlegm can be considered as a kind of food supply for the body.
- Maintaining or improving flexibility is owed to the humor of phlegm, so very much like other humors phlegm is of great benefits to the body.

Excessive Phlegm Symptoms

- Feeling heavy specially the eyelids and the head, getting puffy and swollen, feeling cold (in contrast with people with sanguine temperament), breaking into cold sweat, getting sweaty palms, getting pale, not feeling thirsty or feeling false thirst, increased mucus production (getting runny nose or watery eyes), stringy or thick saliva, weakness, weakened muscle, sagging of skin, sleepiness, having trouble waking up especially in dam places or northern cities with high humidity and during cold seasons, memory loss, dizziness, difficulty learning or remembering something, having difficulty digesting food, bloating, frequent urination, sour burp, and diarrhea are the symptoms of excessive phlegm in the body.

- On the other hand, joint making cracking sounds can be a symptom of lack of phlegm. Joints, respiratory and digestive tract would function healthily with sufficient amounts of phlegm.

Phlegm Producing Foods

- Food that look like water or have similar characteristics as water by being odorless, tasteless, colorless, and food that are watery and slimy such as soups, broths, and sour stews containing vegetables, water from boiled Kaleh pache (dish of boiled cow or sheep's feet and/or head) or tripe (edible lining from the stomachs of sheep), frozen food, raw food, or cooked food served cold, consuming too much rice without bran, potato, tomato, sauces particularly mayonnaise, salads, dairy products, water, fruits and vegetables with cold Mizaj (cooling characteristics) such as lettuce, cucumber, citrus and sour fruits could form or increase phlegm in the body.

How to Avoid and Treat Excessive Phlegm

- People with excessive phlegm should avoid consuming food that could increase phlegm in the body. Fasting, being hungry and thirsty would benefit such people in that it let them get rid of the excessive phlegm build up in their bodies and become warmer and drier.
- People suffering excessive phlegm should eat low volume, high calorie food stuff such as kebab with small portions of rice and bread, roasted chicken heart for a week, bird meat like quail and partridge, toasted nuts (in general toasting, stir frying, and sautéing food stuff is good for such people), dried fig, raisin, dried berries, rock candy, honey, natural sweets, one tea spoon of date and grape syrup a day, sweet homemade jams, fairly salty food with spices such as pepper, cinnamon, cardamom, vegetables such as mint, leek, tarragon, parsley and savory as well as fruits like ripen and sweet apple, mango, banana, and pear.

CHUMASH TRADITIONAL MEDICINE

Chumash traditional medicine is a type of traditional medicine practiced by the Chumash people of the southern coastal regions of California.

Chumash medicine focused on treating mind, spirit, and body alike to promote the wellness of both the individual and the larger community. Healing practices included a knowledge of local plants, as well as a mix of spiritual practices including prayer, singing, and dancing. Post-European contact, Chumash healers adapted these methods to treat changes in environment and the introduction of deadly diseases. Prevention was key in promoting health, and healers took responsibility for ensuring all people worked and felt valued in the community. In the modern day, certain medicinal practices are viewed as controversial, including the treatment of menstruating women, the use of sacred datura, and the consumption of dangerous polycyclic aromatic hydrocarbons.

Herbalism

List of Chumash Medicinal Herbs

The climate of the Chumash territory supported a variety of plant species, many of which were used in medicine. The following list provides a sampling of commonly used plants in Chumash healing practices, but cannot be considered complete.

Similarity to Chinese Herbalism

Certain aspects of Chumash healing practices have been compared to those used in Chinese healing. The use of certain healing touches, as well as spiritual practices in healing are well-documented in both cultures. Notably, plants of the same genus were often used to achieve the same healing effect. For example, the poppies *papaver californicum* in California and *papaver somniferum* were used to treat pain. Both species contain morphine and papaverine, powerful opiates. Several other medicinal parallels between the two cultures exist, including the use of diterpenoids and flavones to treat skin irritations and flavonols and tannins for diarrhea.

Spiritual Foundations

Both medical philosophies rely on maintaining the balance between two forces, the Yin and Yang for the Chinese, and the Sun and Sky Coyote for the Chumash. In Chinese practice, Yin is the inhibiting force, while Yang is the activating. The Sun and Sky Coyote personify the dualistic philosophy of the Chumash, with a hot and unforgiving Sun, and a cool and generous Sky. In both traditions, balance must be maintained to achieve good health, and treatment for illness usually looks to fortify whichever side is lacking, as determined by a trained healer. This duality is represented in divisions of day and night, male and female, and hot and cold, among others. The Chinese treat diseases caused by cold with plant remedies which warm the patient, such as those with adrenergic properties which increase heart rate and blood flow. Chumash peoples bathe daily in cold water, but use sweat lodges and hot springs to harness the healing powers of heat.

Cross-cultural Contact

Some historians argue that Chinese peoples landed in California in the early 15th century, but the validity of such claims remain in dispute. However, it is more likely that Polynesian peoples had contact with both the Chinese and indigenous nations in California, potentially facilitating the transfer of herbal knowledge. Still some maintain that humans innately look to plants as potential medicines, and only those groups which successfully utilize plants are able to survive.

Spiritualism in Healing

For the Chumash people, spiritual practices played an equally important role as medicinal plants in the healing process. Body, mind, and spirit were seen as indistinguishable, so treatments had to account for all aspects of the self to be effective. The first remedies focused on the spiritual to open the mind and body to healing.

In Chumash culture, the most important work of the Healer occurred before anyone fell ill. Obesity was virtually non-existent, largely due to diet and a culture which did not tolerate laziness, seen to lead to excessive weight gain. By working all day, the Chumash kept physically fit, reducing the prevalence of heart disease and high blood pressure, and the feeling of being needed by the community was thought to help strengthen the spirit. Additionally, it was common for the Chumash to bathe regularly, promoting good hygiene habits and warding off disease. Healers regularly encouraged these practices, and they themselves practiced routing fasting and prayer to strengthen their spirits.

Before treating a patient, the Healer began with prayer, to invite the participation of God (Xoy in Chumash) in the healing process. A patient may lie beside a fire, so they can be comforted by the warmth and sound of the flames. Healing is also a communal process, and the patient may be joined by family and friends dancing, singing, fasting, and praying around them, and offering them emotional support. To start, white sage is burned in a seashell to strengthen the spirit and help calm the patient, keeping them in a rational, coherent state. The shell is moved so as to allow the smoke to touch all parts of the patient. Small amounts of momoy may be given to those who do not listen well, or have domineering personalities, to help them relax. Humor is another valuable tool for the Healer to relieve anxieties and allow the patient's spirit a chance to heal.

Women's Health

Chumash women were respected as life-bringers and nurturers of family and community. As such, there was a variety of practices and treatments to help them through menstruation, childbirth, lactation, and menopause.

Menstruation

Women were kept isolated during menstruation and prohibited from eating meat or drinking cold water for three days. They also could not bathe, despite daily bathing being common in Chumash culture. Instead, they used the leaves of Wooly Bluecurls as douches. White sage was used to control heavy bleeding. Dysmenorrhea and premenstrual syndrome were treated with mugwort or Paeonia californica. Many treatments could be harmful in large doses.

Urinary Tract Infection

Urinary tract infections were treated with teas meant to increase urination and raise the pH of the urine, creating a hostile environment for bacteria. Teas could be made from Ephedra viridis or Ephedra californica, as well as corn silk.

Childbirth

If possible, childbirth took place in a special hut under the guidance of a midwife, though it was not uncommon for pregnant women to give birth on their own if they were too far from the village. Mugwort was burned to be used as aromatherapy to ease labor pains. Trichostema lanatum and Trichostema lanceolatum also relieved pain and was used to facilitate delivery of the afterbirth. These plants could then be used as a douche. The umbilical cord was cut with a knife made from carrizo cane and ash was spread on the infant's navel to stop the bleeding.

After giving birth, women bathed in cold water. Husbands were prohibited from touching their wives after childbirth until that child could walk on its own.

Venereal Diseases

Gonorrhea afflicted the Chumash people pre-European contact, but cases of the disease increased with the rise of Spanish missions, decreasing fertility. Rock powder was believed to increase fertility. Yerba mansa was believed to cure gonorrhea, as well as many other afflictions. Seawater was used to treat sores from venereal diseases, as well as tea made from carrizo cane.

Controversial Practices

Polycyclic Aromatic Hydrocarbon Consumption

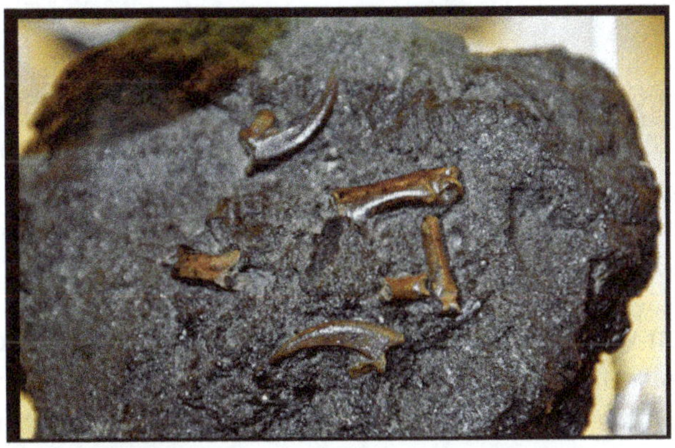

Fossil bird bones and talons in tar, found in Kern County, California. Similar to that encountered by Chumash Indians.

Polycyclic aromatic hydrocarbons (PAHs) are a chemical product of fossil fuels, found in substances such as gasoline, tar, and cigarettes. The adverse health effects of PAHs are well-researched, perversely affecting the human body via the nervous system, hormonal disruptions, and fetal abnormalities.

Before the industrial era, the predominant form of PAHs was found in natural bitumen from fossils. One of the most concentrated regions of bitumen in the world is the region home to the Chumash, where they used bitumen in myriad materials, including tomol canoes and water-carrying baskets. Thus, the Chumash have been a target of interest for research on PAH exposure, owing to their prolific use of PAH-containing bitumen over the previous millennia (with evidence of use in objects as far back as 10,000 years ago).

Wärmländer et al. have studied the skeletons of Chumash between 6500 BCE and the beginning of significant European contact (mid-1700s) and found a number of consistent decreases in Chumash health over the time of bitumen use. Among these markers was systematic decreases in skull size for both males and females over the studied timescale, indicating both decreased birthweight and neurological development over millennia. Despite that these adverse health outcomes are consistent with PAH exposure, some argue that a direct link between bitumen use and decreased Chumash health is still not known. Patricia Lambert of Utah State University is among Chumash experts who question the hypothesis of bitumen use leading to poorer Chumash health, citing the need for increased research on the controversial topic.

Cancer Prevention and Remedy

Among the problems associated with PAH exposure is increased incidence of cancers. Thus, a number of Chumash methods have been developed to deal with cancer management. As discussed, spiritual practices were integral to Chumash medicinal practices. This included the use of hallucinogenic substances, along with techniques such as hypnosis though chanting, as practiced by other Native American populations. It is also hypothesized that a number of plants consumed by the Chumash may have alleviated the harmful effects of PAH exposure, leading to modern theories about botanical and nutritive cancer-prevention substances. Once again, this is where Chumash and Native medicinal practice reaches an impasse with much of modern Western medicine. It is thus a topic of controversy among Chumash researchers and medical professionals.

Sacred Datura

Datura, also called "momoy" by the Chumash or "jimsonweed", is a hallucinogenic plant commonly consumed as a liquid in traditional Chumash spiritual practice. Early anthropological records indicate adolescent males and females would receive datura from a "giver" when seemed ready for its rite of passage. Typically, Chumash restrictions on diet and sex would be observed by individuals before ingestion.

The effects of datura often would consist of up to a day of incapacitation, the length of which was viewed to indicate the spiritual strength of the individual. Hallucinations in dreams and of animals such as hawks or coyotes were viewed as marks of a successful datura experience. The effects of datura, however, vary greatly by dosage, and current understanding indicates lasting adverse physiological effects up to days to months after ingestion.

The most significant side-effect of datura can be death, as the lethal dose of the drug is very slightly more than the necessary dose to produce hallucinations. Deaths from datura in Chumash communities were often seen as the fault of the drinker, who was assumed to deviate from the necessary dietary or sexual restrictions or have chosen to not come back from the experience. For this reason, the use of datura has been criticized by many for being too dangerous, especially as its use is often begun in adolescence.

UNANI MEDICINE

Unani or Yunani medicine is the pseudoscientific practice used in Perso-Arabic traditional medicine in Mughal India and in Muslim culture in South Asia and modern day Central Asia.

The Hellenistic origin of Unani medicine is still visible in its being based on the classical four humours: phlegm (balgham), blood (dam), yellow bile (Ṣafrā) and black bile (saudā'), but it has also been influenced by Indian and Chinese traditional systems.

According to Unani medicine, management of any disease depends upon the diagnosis of disease. Proper diagnosis depends upon observation of the patient's symptoms and temperament.

Unani, like Ayurveda, is based on theory of the presence of the elements in the human body. According to followers of Unani medicine, these elements are present in fluids and their balance leads to health and their imbalance leads to illness.

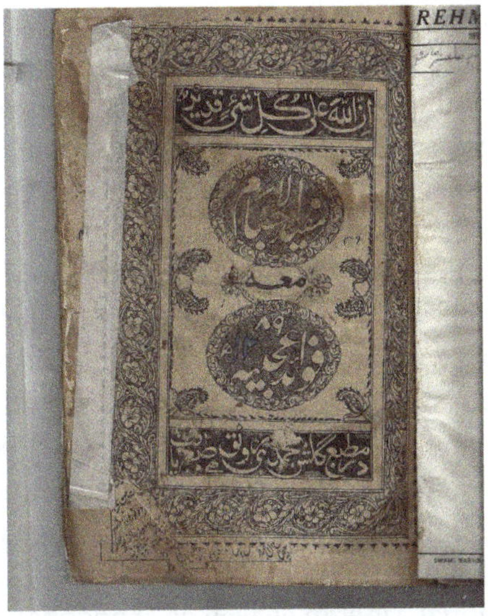

A title page of Unani book on physiology in Urdu.

According to Unani practitioners, the failure of the Quwwat-e-Mudabbira-e-Badan, or the body's ability to maintain its own health, may lead to derangement of the normal equilibrium of the body's akhlat (humors). Abnormal humors are believed to lead to pathological changes in the tissues at the affected site, creating the clinical manifestations of illness. The theory postulates the presence of blood, phlegm, yellow bile and black bile in the human body. Each person's unique mixture of these substances determines his mizaj (temperament). A predominance of blood gives a sanguine temperament; a predominance of phlegm makes one phlegmatic; yellow bile, bilious (or choleric); and black bile, melancholic.

After diagnosing the disease, treatment follows a pattern (*Usool-e-ilaj*):

- Izalae Sabab (elimination of cause).
- Tadeele Akhlat (normalization of humors).
- Tadeele Aza (normalization of tissues/organs).

Treatment includes regimens and therapies included in the term *Ilaj-Bil-Tadbeer*. These therapies include cupping, aromatherapy, bloodletting, bathing, exercise, and *dalak* (massaging the body). It may also involve the prescription of Unani drugs or surgery.

Unani products like egg oil and almond oil are commonly used for hair care in India, and registered Unani practitioners are treated as qualified doctors in India and Pakistan.

TRADITIONAL MONGOLIAN MEDICINE

Traditional Mongolian Medicine represents an Asian medical tradition which is greatly) to (by the Mongols.

Traditional healing methods of non-European societies, mainly of Asian origin, have become more popular in the West during the past decades. The spreading of knowledge about traditional medicines is due to various factors such as growing tourism, publicity in the worldwide web, traditional treatments applied by Asian physicians touring the West and the increasing demand of Western patients for alternative or complementary therapy. Traditional Chinese medicine (TCM), Ayurveda, Kampo and Traditional Tibetan Medicine represent the better known traditional systems. Rather unknown to the public is the traditional medicine of the Mongolian people. Based on Mongolian folk medicine, Traditional Mongolian Medicine had developed by replacing many shamanistic practices with medical theories, techniques and medication of Traditional Tibetan Medicine. The Mongolian medical system also integrated some aspects of other oriental medicines such as Ayurveda and Chinese medicine. Traditional Tibetan Medicine was introduced to the Mongols in the 16th century when Lamaism became the leading religion. For centuries, Tibetan Buddhism had influenced the daily life and the religious practice of the Mongolians as well as the medical education of the Mongolian physicians. Monks were educated in traditional medicine in the monasteries and played an important role in the health system of the past. Medical disputations and the exchange of ideas between Mongolian and Tibetan doctors stimulated the development of the medical system on both sides. The term "emchi" which is used to address a traditional Tibetan as well as Mongolian physician is actually the Mongolian word for "medical doctor".

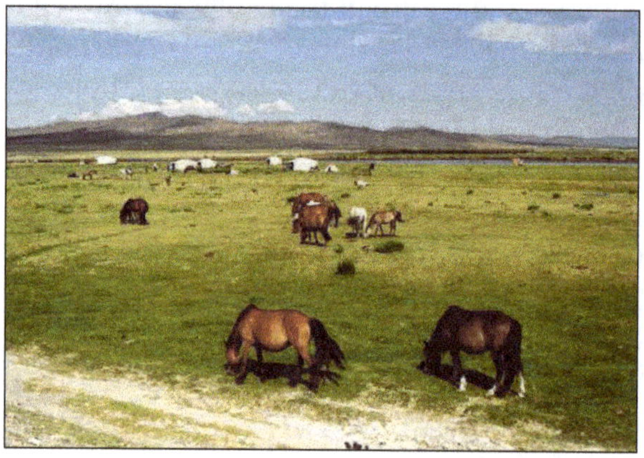

Landscape with traditional nomadic dwellings.

The Khalkha Mongols are the main ethnic group of the Republic of Mongolia representing almost 82% of the about 2.59 million inhabitants. The Buryats are another large ethnic group of Mongolian descent, who live in Siberia, mainly in the Republic of Buryatia. They represent 436 000 citizens of the Russian Federation. In China, 5.8 million Mongols of different Mongolian ethnic groups are counted. The majority of those Mongolians, 3.5 million, live in the Inner Mongolia Autonomous Region.

Principles of Traditional Mongolian Medicine

The basics of Traditional Mongolian Medicine follow mainly the guidelines of Tibetan medicine and Tibetan Buddhism. There exists a great variety of ancient medical treatises written by Mongolian authors as well as Mongolian translations of renowned Tibetan medical books. Until today, Mongolian traditional doctors accept the main Tibetan medical treatise, the rgyud bzhi, as the basis of their medical knowledge. According to traditional medicine the human body is understood as an entity. Human health relies on the equilibrium of the three life-sustaining principles, named in Mongolian hii (Tibetan rlung), šar (Tibetan mkhris pa) and badgan (Tibetan bad kan). These terms are often translated into English as wind (hii), bile (šar) and phlegm (badgan), but they should not be confused with the same English terms used in antique Greek medicine. Any disturbance in the equilibrium of the three principles results in a disease. Therefore, re-establishing the equilibrium in the patient's body is the foremost task of the traditional physician. In general, hot and cold disorders are differentiated in Traditional Mongolian Medicine. To diagnose a disease the traditional physician reads the pulses, examines the tongue, checks the urine by smell, colour and taste and interrogates the patient. However, pulse reading is the main traditional diagnostic tool, because the physician checks the type of the disease (hot or cold) and the conditions of the internal organs in this way. He must be well experienced in recognising the healthy pulse in order to differentiate it from the pulse which indicates a specific disease. Consequently, the traditionally diagnosed disorders do not easily match diseases as diagnosed by Western medicine. However, some symptoms listed in the traditional texts relate to Western disease syndromes.

The therapy of disease, according to traditional medicine, focuses first on changes in the patient's diet and behaviour in daily life. Other therapeutic measures are medication, massages, blood-letting, steam baths, drinking of mineral water, acupuncture and moxibustion. Moxibustion refers to a specific treatment. A cone made up of a powdered plant is stuck to a specific point of the body. Then, the cone is lightened to burn down slowly warming up the respective part of the body. The medical preparations used to cure the disorders are complex mixtures of a varying number of ingredients, mainly plants, but they contain also minerals and animal drugs such as musk or sheep's liver. In general, one ingredient of a medicine is always specified as the leading one while the remaining ones support the main ingredient in its efficacy. A specific nature (cooling, warming and neutral) and particular qualities and secondary qualities which influence the three life-sustaining principles in the body are assigned to each ingredient.

Taste, property, qualities and secondary qualities of medicinal plants according to Traditional Mongolian Medicine

Plant Species / Family	Taste	Property	Quality	Secondary Quality
Dianthus versicolor Fisch./ Caryophyllaceae	bitter	cooling	cool	coarse
				blunt
				light
Gentiana barbata Froel./ Gentianaceae	bitter	cooling	cool	coarse
				blunt
Gentiana decumbens L. f./ Gentianaceae	bitter, astringent	cooling	cool	smooth
				Flexible
				Fluidity
Lilum pumilum DC./ Liliaceae	sweet	cooling	Cool	Cool
Myricaria longifolia Ehrenb./ Tamaricaceae	astringent, bitter	cooling	Cool	heavy
			blunt	stable
Saussurea amara L. (DC)/ Asteraceae	bitter	cooling	light	coarse
				blunt

In general, hot diseases are treated with medicines having mainly a cooling nature, while cold diseases require a treatment with medicines of a warming nature. The efficacy of a medicinal product greatly depends on the proper blending of the ingredients according to their inherent qualities in order to achieve a stimulation of the healing process. A hot disease requires another blending of the ingredient's qualities than a cold disease. Therefore, it is very important that the qualities and secondary qualities of the ingredients are well-balanced, because otherwise the medicine may exert an adverse effect on the patient instead of a favourable one.

In the past the traditional physician collected the necessary plants, minerals and animal products for his medication on his own in his living area and bought missing drugs at the markets, sometimes in distant places. The basic information about medication and the characteristics for identifying the plants, minerals and animal drugs is found in the traditional medical texts. However, to identify the ingredients the physicians rely on different oral traditions and written documentaries laid down by renowned scholars of the past. Consequently, differences in the identification of the plants, animal drugs and minerals produce different ingredients. Moreover, regarding plants, differences in the vegetation of different collection areas lead to the harvesting of different plant species. Therefore, the same Mongolian plant name may stand for more than one species and different plants may be collected under the same traditional name. In the past, each traditional physician prepared the medicine for his patients himself according to the prescriptions of the medical texts or his own experiences. Today, the mode of preparing medicines has greatly changed. A large amount of the traditional medicines is now produced in the big centres of traditional medicine as well as by Mongolian companies using modern production methods. The needed plants, animal drugs and minerals are collected by the locals in the Mongolian countryside or the ingredients are purchased at various markets in and outside Mongolia. Such prefabricated traditional medicines are sold within the Republic of Mongolia, some of the products are even exported. Legal regulations are issued to control drug identity, efficacy and safety.

References

- Mirghazanfari, Seyyed Mahdi (2017-05-24). "Iranian traditional medicine prioritizes health maintenance over treatment". Tehran Times. Retrieved 2018-05-14
- De las Peñas, César Fernández; Arendt-Nielsen, Lars; Gerwin, Robert D (2010). Tension-type and cervicogenic headache: pathophysiology, diagnosis, and management. Jones & Bartlett Learning. Pp. 251–254. ISBN 9780763752835
- Traditional-Chinese-medicine, science: britannica.com, Retrieved 5 February, 2019
- Selin, Helaine (2013-11-11). Encyclopaedia of the History of Science, Technology, and Medicine in Non-Western Cultures. Springer Science & Business Media. P. 506. ISBN 9789401714167. Retrieved 9 September2016
- Adams JD, Garcia C (March 2006). "Women's health among the Chumash". Evidence-Based Complementary and Alternative Medicine. 3 (1): 125–31. Doi:10.1093/ecam/nek021. PMC 1375244. PMID 16550233
- Timbrook J (2007). Chumash Ethnobotany: Plant Knowledge Among the Chumash People of Southern California. Santa Barbara, Calif.: Santa Barbara Museum of Natural History. ISBN 978-1-59714-048-5
- Justice RK Agrawal (13 April 2018). "Judgment by the Supreme Court of India: Kerala Ayurveda Paramparya vs State Of Kerala". Supreme Court of India. Retrieved 9 December 2019

Ayurveda

3 CHAPTER

Ayurveda is a type of alternative medicine which was developed in the Indian subcontinent. It has eight major branches namely kaaya chikitsa, baala chikitsa, graha chikitsa, urdhaanga chikitsa, shalyaroga chikitsa, damstra chikitsa, jara tantra and vajikarana. The topics elaborated in this chapter will help in gaining a better perspective about these branches of Ayurveda.

Ayurveda is considered by many scholars to be the oldest healing science. Ayurvedic knowledge originated in India more than 5,000 years ago and is often called the "Mother of All Healing." It stems from the ancient Vedic culture and was taught for many thousands of years in an oral tradition from accomplished masters to their disciples. Some of this knowledge was set to print a few thousand years ago, but much of it is inaccessible. The principles of many of the natural healing systems now familiar in the West have their roots in Ayurveda, including Homeopathy and Polarity Therapy.

The Strategy

Your Constitution and its Inner Balance

Ayurveda places great emphasis on prevention and encourages the maintenance of health through close attention to balance in one's life, right thinking, diet, lifestyle and the use of herbs. Knowledge of Ayurveda enables one to understand how to create this balance of body, mind and consciousness according to one's own individual constitution and how to make lifestyle changes to bring about and maintain this balance. Just as everyone has a unique fingerprint, each person has a particular pattern of energy—an individual combination of physical, mental and emotional characteristics—which comprises their own constitution. This constitution is determined at conception by a number of factors and remains the same throughout one's life.

Many factors, both internal and external, act upon us to disturb this balance and are reflected as a change in one's constitution from the balanced state. Examples of these emotional and physical stresses include one's emotional state, diet and food choices, seasons and weather, physical trauma, work and family relationships. Once these factors are understood, one can take appropriate actions to nullify or minimize their effects or eliminate the causes of imbalance and re-establish one's original constitution. Balance is the natural order; imbalance is disorder. Health is order; disease is disorder. Within the body there is a constant interaction between order and disorder. When one understands the nature and structure of disorder, one can re-establish order.

Balancing the three Principle Energies of the Body

Ayurveda identifies three basic types of energy or functional principles that are present in everyone and everything. Since there are no single words in English that convey these concepts, we use the original Sanskrit words vata, pitta and kapha. These principles can be related to the basic biology of the body.

Energy is required to create movement so that fluids and nutrients get to the cells, enabling the body to function. Energy is also required to metabolize the nutrients in the cells, and is called for to lubricate and maintain the structure of the cell. Vata is the energy of movement; pitta is the energy of digestion or metabolism and kapha, the energy of lubrication and structure. All people have the qualities of vata, pitta and kapha, but one is usually primary, one secondary and the third is usually least prominent. The cause of disease in Ayurveda is viewed as a lack of proper cellular function due to an excess or deficiency of vata, pitta or kapha. Disease can also be caused by the presence of toxins.

In Ayurveda, body, mind and consciousness work together in maintaining balance. They are simply viewed as different facets of one's being. To learn how to balance the body, mind and consciousness requires an understanding of how vata, pitta and kapha work together. According to Ayurvedic philosophy the entire cosmos is an interplay of the energies of the five great elements—Space, Air, Fire, Water and Earth. Vata, pitta and kapha are combinations and permutations of these five elements that manifest as patterns present in all creation. In the physical body, vata is the subtle energy of movement, pitta the energy of digestion and metabolism, and kapha the energy that forms the body's structure.

Vata is the subtle energy associated with movement — composed of Space and Air. It governs breathing, blinking, muscle and tissue movement, pulsation of the heart, and all movements in the cytoplasm and cell membranes. In balance, vata promotes creativity and flexibility. Out of balance, vata produces fear and anxiety.

Pitta expresses as the body's metabolic system — made up of Fire and Water. It governs digestion, absorption, assimilation, nutrition, metabolism and body temperature. In balance, pitta promotes understanding and intelligence. Out of balance, pitta arouses anger, hatred and jealousy.

Kapha is the energy that forms the body's structure — bones, muscles, tendons — and provides the "glue" that holds the cells together, formed from Earth and Water. Kapha supplies the water for all bodily parts and systems. It lubricates joints, moisturizes the skin, and maintains immunity. In balance, kapha is expressed as love, calmness and forgiveness. Out of balance, it leads to attachment, greed and envy.

Life presents us with many challenges and opportunities. Although there is much over which we have little control, we do have the power to decide about some things, such as diet and lifestyle. To maintain balance and health, it is important to pay attention to these decisions. Diet and lifestyle appropriate to one's individual constitution strengthen the body, mind and consciousness.

Ayurveda as a Complementary System of Healing

The basic difference between Ayurveda and Western allopathic medicine is important to understand. Western allopathic medicine currently tends to focus on symptomatology and disease, and primarily uses drugs and surgery to rid the body of pathogens or diseased tissue. Many lives have been saved by this approach. In fact, surgery is encompassed by Ayurveda. However, drugs, because of their toxicity, often weaken the body. Ayurveda does not focus on disease. Rather, Ayurveda maintains that all life must be supported by energy in balance. When there is minimal stress and the flow of energy within a person is balanced, the body's natural defense systems will be strong and can more easily defend against disease.

It must be emphasized that Ayurveda is not a substitute for Western allopathic medicine. There are many instances when the disease process and acute conditions can best be treated with drugs or surgery. Ayurveda can be used in conjunction with Western medicine to make a person stronger and less likely to be afflicted with disease and/or to rebuild the body after being treated with drugs or surgery.

We all have times when we don't feel well and recognize that we're out of balance. Sometimes we go to the doctor only to be told there is nothing wrong. What is actually occurring is that this imbalance has not yet become recognizable as a disease. Yet it is serious enough to make us notice our discomfort. We may start to wonder whether it is just our imagination. We may also begin to consider alternative measures and actively seek to create balance in our body, mind and consciousness.

Evaluation and Treatment of Imbalances

Ayurveda encompasses various techniques for assessing health. The practitioner carefully evaluates key signs and symptoms of illness, especially in relation to the origin and cause of an imbalance. They also consider the patient's suitability for various treatments. The practitioner arrives at diagnosis through direct questioning, observation and a physical exam, as well as inference. Basic techniques such taking the pulse, observing the tongue, eyes and physical form; and listening to the tone of the voice are employed during an assessment.

Palliative and cleansing measures, when appropriate, can be used to help eliminate an imbalance along with suggestions for eliminating or managing the causes of the imbalance. Recommendations may include the implementation of lifestyle changes; starting and maintaining a suggested diet; and the use of herbs. In some cases, participating in a cleansing program, called panchakarma, is suggested to help the body rid itself of accumulated toxins to gain more benefit from the various suggested measures of treatment.

Ayurveda addresses all aspects of life — the body, mind and spirit. It recognizes that each of us is unique, each responds differently to the many aspects of life, each possesses different strengths and weaknesses. Through insight, understanding and experience Ayurveda presents a vast wealth of information on the relationships between causes and their effects, both immediate and subtle, for each unique individual.

Vata

The Energy of Movement

Vata provides the essential motion for all bodily processes and is extremely vital for health. On an annual basis, vāta is most prominent in the fall and at the change of seasons, and these are the most important times to be careful of diet and lifestyle. One purpose of lifestyle considerations is stabilize this motion. Routine is very useful in assisting the vata individual to effectively ground all this moving energy.

A person with vata predominant is blessed with a quick mind, flexibility and creativity. Mentally, they usually grasp concepts quickly but then forget them just as quickly. Alert, restless and very active, vata people walk, talk and think fast, but are easily fatigued. They tend to have less willpower, confidence, boldness and tolerance for fluctuation than other types and often feel unstable and ungrounded. When unbalanced, vata types may become fearful, nervous and anxious. In the external world, vata types tend to earn money quickly and spend it quickly. They are not good planners and as a consequence may suffer economic hardship.

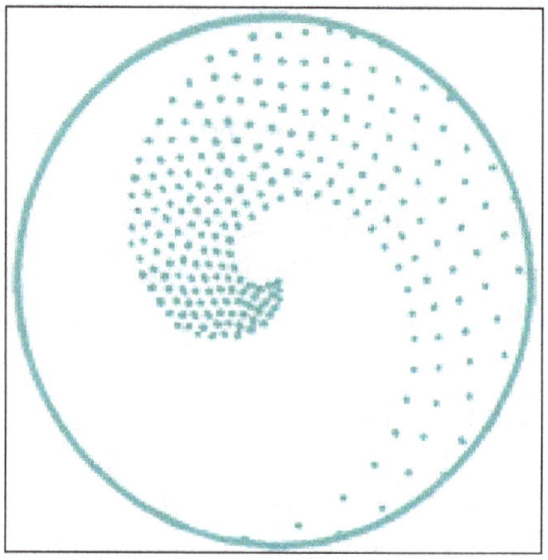

Vata types have variable appetite and digestion. They are often attracted to astringent foods like salad and raw vegetables, but their constitution is balanced by warm, cooked foods and sweet, sour and salty tastes. With a tendency to produce little urine, their feces are often hard, dry and small in size and quantity.

Vata resides in the colon, as well as the brain, ears, bones, joints, skin and thighs. Vata people are more susceptible to diseases involving the air principle, such as emphysema, pneumonia and arthritis. Other common vata disorders include flatulence, tics, twitches, aching joints, dry skin and hair, nerve disorders, constipation, and mental confusion. Vata in the body tends to increase with age as is exhibited by the drying and wrinkling of the skin.

Since the attributes of vata are dry, light, cold, rough, subtle, mobile and clear, any of these qualities in excess can cause imbalance. Frequent travel, especially by plane, loud noises, continual stimulation, drugs, sugar and alcohol all derange vata, as does exposure to cold and cold liquids and foods. Like the wind, vata types have a hard time becoming and staying grounded. Routine is difficult but essential if vata is to be lowered and controlled. It is best for vata types to go to bed by 10 PM as they need more rest than the other types. In general, people with excessive vata respond most rapidly to warm, moist, slightly oily, heavy foods. Steam baths, humidifiers and moisture in general are helpful. Daily oil massage before bath or shower is also recommended.

Dietary Considerations

General food guidelines for decreasing vata include warm, well-cooked, unctuous foods. One should have small meals three or four times a day and may snack as needed while maintaining a two hour gap between each meal. Regularity in meal times is important for vata. Those with vata-dominant constitutions do well with one- pot meals such as soups, stews and casseroles. They can use more oil in cooking their foods than the other two doshas and experience better digestion if they limit their intake of raw foods.

Well-cooked oats and rice are good for vata because they are not too drying when cooked with plenty of water and butter or ghee. While cooked vegetables are best for vata, the occasional salad with a good oily or creamy dressing is all right. Nightshades—tomatoes, potatoes, eggplants and peppers—as well as spinach should be avoided if the vata person has stiff, aching joints or muscles. Sweet, ripe and juicy fruits are good for vata. The astringent and drying fruits, such as cranberries, pomegranates and raw apples, should be avoided. Fruit should always be eaten by itself on an empty stomach.

Many vata people can satisfy their need for protein by judicious use of dairy products, but can also use eggs, chicken, turkey, fresh fish and venison if they wish. Legumes are difficult to digest and should be consumed in limited quantity by those trying to pacify vata. The legumes should be the split type and soaked before cooking. Cooking them with a little oil and spices, such as turmeric, cumin, coriander, ginger, garlic and hing (asafoetida), will help prevent vata from being disturbed.

All nuts and seeds are good for vata, but are best used as butters or milks. Ten almonds, soaked in water overnight with skins removed the next morning, are a satisfying early morning food. Sesame oil is warming for vata, but all oils are good. All dairy products are good for vata with hard cheese being eaten sparingly. All spices are good, but should not be overused. Vatas can have half a glass of wine, diluted with water, during or after a meal. Since vata people tend to be prone to addiction, they should avoid sugar, caffeine and tobacco. Intensity itself can be intoxicating to vata, so one should seek relaxation and meditation to reduce vata.

General guidelines for balancing vata:

- Keep warm,
- Keep calm,
- Avoid cold, frozen or raw foods,
- Avoid extreme cold,
- Eat warm foods and spices,
- Keep a regular routine,
- Get plenty of rest.

Pitta

The Energy of Digestion and Metabolism

Pitta types have many of the qualities of fire. Fire is hot, penetrating, sharp and agitating. Similarly, pitta people have warm bodies, penetrating ideas and sharp intelligence. When out of balance, they can become very agitated and short-tempered. The pitta body type is one of medium height and build, with ruddy or coppery skin. They may have many moles and freckles. Their skin is warm and less wrinkled than vata skin. Their hair tends to be silky and they often experience premature graying or hair loss. Their eyes are of medium size and the conjunctiva is moist. The nose is sharp and the tip tends to be reddish.

Those with pitta-dominant constitutions have a strong metabolism, good digestion and strong appetites. They like plenty of food and liquids and tend to love hot spices and cold drinks. However, their constitution is balanced by sweet, bitter and astringent tastes. Pitta people's sleep is sound and of medium duration. They produce large quantities of urine and feces, which tend to be yellowish, soft and plentiful. They perspire easily and their hands and feet stay warm. Pitta people have a lower tolerance for sunlight, heat and hard physical work.

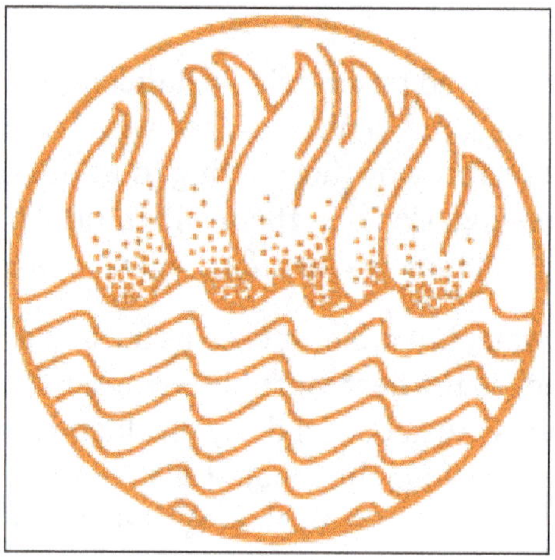

Mentally, pitta types are alert and intelligent and have good powers of comprehension. However, they are easily agitated and aggressive and tend toward hate, anger and jealousy when imbalanced. In the external world, pitta people like to be leaders and planners and seek material prosperity. They like to exhibit their wealth and possessions. Pitta people tend to have diseases involving the fire principle such as fevers, inflammatory diseases and jaundice. Common symptoms include skin rashes, burning sensation, ulceration, fever, inflammations or irritations such as conjunctivitis, colitis or sore throats.

Since the attributes of pitta are oily, hot, light, mobile, dispersing and liquid, an excess of any of these qualities aggravates pitta. Summer is a time of heat, the pitta season. Sunburn, poison ivy, prickly heat and short tempers are common. These kinds of pitta disorders tend to calm down as the weather gets cooler. The diet and lifestyle changes emphasize coolness—cool foods, avoidance of chilies and spices (especially difficult for New Mexicans), and cool climates. People with excessive pitta need to exercise at the coolest part of the day.

Dietary Considerations

General food guidelines for pacifying pitta include avoiding sour, salty and pungent foods. Vegetarianism is best for pitta people and they should refrain from eating meat, eggs, alcohol and salt. To help calm their natural aggressiveness and compulsiveness, it is beneficial to incorporate sweet, cooling and bitter foods and tastes into their diets.

Barley, rice, oats and wheat are good grains for pitta dominant individuals and vegetables should form a substantial part of their diet. Tomatoes, radishes, chilies, garlic and raw onions should all be avoided. In fact, any vegetable that is too sour or hot will aggravate pitta, but most other vegetables will help to calm it. Daikon radishes are cleansing for the liver when pitta is in balance but should be avoided otherwise. Salads and raw vegetables are good for pitta types in the spring and summer as are any sweet fruits. Sour fruits should be avoided with the exception of limes, used sparingly.

Animal foods, especially seafood and eggs, should only be taken in moderation by pitta types. Chicken, turkey, rabbit and venison are all right. All legumes except red and yellow lentils are good in small amounts, with black lentils, chickpeas and mung beans being the best.

Most nuts and seeds have too much oil and are heating for pitta. However, coconut is cooling and sunflower and pumpkin seeds are all right occasionally. Small amounts of coconut, olive and sunflower oils are also good for pitta.

Sweet dairy products are good and include milk, unsalted butter, ghee and soft, unsalted cheeses. Yogurt can be used if it is blended with spices, a little sweetener and water. In fact, pitta people can use a sweetener better than the other two doshas because it relieves pitta. However, they should avoid hot spices, using cardamom, cinnamon, coriander, fennel and turmeric predominantly, with small amounts of cumin and black pepper.

Coffee, alcohol and tobacco should be completely avoided although the occasional beer may be relaxing for a pitta person. Black tea may also be used occasionally with a little milk and a pinch of cardamom.

General guidelines for balancing pitta:

- Avoid excessive heat.
- Avoid excessive oil.
- Avoid excessive steam.
- Limit salt intake.
- Eat cooling, non-spicy foods.
- Exercise during the cooler part of the day.

Kapha

The Energy of Lubrication

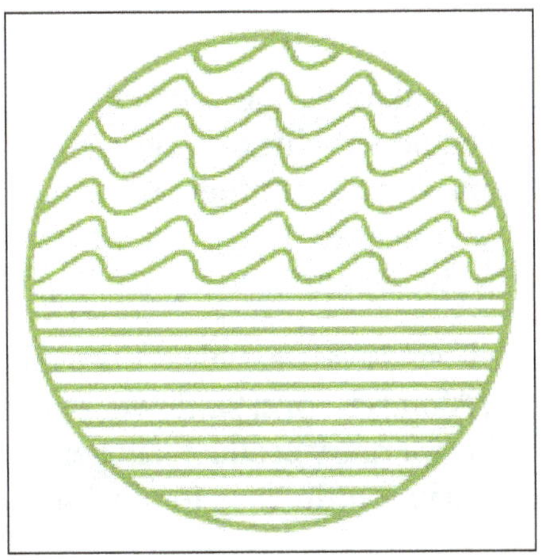

Kapha types are blessed with strength, endurance and stamina. In balance, they tend to have sweet, loving dispositions and be stable and grounded. Their skin is oily and smooth. Physically, kapha people may gain weight easily and have a slow metabolism. They tend to shun exercise. They have thick skin and their bodies and muscles are well developed. Their eyes are large and attractive with thick, long lashes and brows. Kapha people evacuate slowly and feces tend to be soft, pale and oily. Perspiration is moderate. Sleep is deep and prolonged. Kapha types are attracted to sweet, salty and oily foods, but their constitutions are most balanced by bitter, astringent and pungent tastes.

Psychologically, kapha people tend to be calm, tolerant and forgiving. However, they may become lethargic. While they may be slow to comprehend, their long term memory is excellent. When out of balance, kaphas tend to experience greed, envy, attachment and possessiveness. In the external world, kapha tendencies toward groundedness, stability and attachment help them to earn and hold onto money.

They are more likely to have diseases connected to the water principle such as flu, sinus congestion, and other diseases involving mucous. Sluggishness, excess weight, diabetes, water retention, and headaches are also common. Kapha can become more aggravated as the moon gets full because there is a tendency for water retention at that time. Winter is the time of greatest kapha accumulation and following the kapha-balancing dietary and lifestyle changes are most important during that season.

Dietary Considerations

Dietary guidelines for kapha people stress bitter, astringent and pungent tastes. They actually need foods that will invigorate their minds while limiting their overall consumption of food. They should avoid dairy products and fats of any kind, especially fried or greasy foods.

Those with kapha dominant constitutions need less grain than pitta or vata constitutions with buckwheat and millet (more heating) being optimal grains for them followed by barley, rice and corn. Roasted or dry cooked grains are best. All vegetables are good for kapha but one should emphasize leafy greens and vegetables grown above ground more than root vegetables while avoiding very sweet, sour or juicy vegetables. Generally kapha people can eat raw vegetables although steamed or stir-fried are easier to digest. Very sweet or sour fruits should be avoided with the more astringent and drying fruits being preferable such as apples, apricots, cranberries, mangoes, peaches and pears.

Only rarely do kapha people need animal foods and, when they do, it should be dry cooked—baked, roasted, boiled—never fried. They could eat chicken, eggs, rabbit, seafood and venison. As their bodies do not require large amounts of protein, they also should not overeat legumes although these are better for them than meat because of the lack of fat. Black beans, mung beans, pinto beans and red lentils are best for kapha types.

The heavy qualities of nuts and seeds aggravate kapha as does the oil in them. Occasional sunflower and pumpkin seeds are all right. Almond, corn, safflower or sunflower oils can be used in small amounts as well. The same holds true for dairy products: in general, kapha people should avoid the heavy, cooling, sweet qualities of dairy. A little ghee for cooking and some consumption of goat's milk is good for kapha types.

Since kapha people should avoid sweets, the only sweetener they should use is raw honey, which is heating. However, they can use all spices, except salt, with ginger and garlic being best for them.

A person whose dominant dosha is kapha and who has very little influence from the other two doshas can benefit from the occasional use of stimulants such as coffee and tea. They are also not as harmed by tobacco and hard liquor. However, they really do not need alcohol at all. If they elect to use alcohol, wine is their best choice.

General guidelines for balancing kapha:

- Get plenty of exercise,
- Avoid heavy foods,
- Keep active,
- Avoid dairy,
- Avoid iced food or drinks,
- Vary your routine,
- Avoid fatty, oily foods,
- Eat light, dry food,
- No daytime naps.

Remember that your progress toward balance and health is proportional to how well you stick to the guidelines of diet and lifestyle. Old habits sometimes die hard and your changes may be very gradual but, to achieve progress, the changes need to be made. You are in charge of your own rate of change.

EIGHT BRANCHES OF AYURVEDA

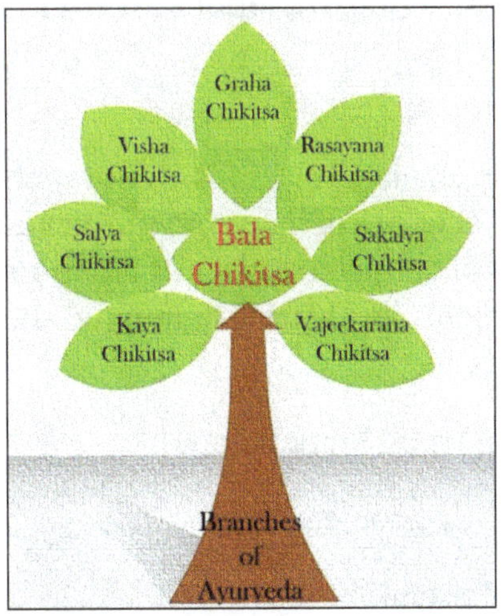

The Eight Branches of Ayurveda are Explained Below:

- Kaaya Chikitsa (Internal medicine).
- Baala Chikitsa (Pediatrics treatment).

- Graha Chikitsa or Bhoot Vidya (Psychiatry).
- Urdhyaanga Chikitsa (Treatment of eyes, nose, throat, head related diseases).
- Shalyaroga Chikitsa (Surgery).
- Damstra Chikitsa – Agad Tantra (Toxicology).
- Jara Chikitsa – Rasayana (Geriatrics).
- Vrishya Chikitsa or Vajjikarana (Aphrodisiac therapy).

Kaaya Chikitsa

Kaaya means "agni" – the digestive fire in the body. It is holistic approach of medicine which is mainly helpful in treatment of whole body. Kaaya Chikitsa is derived from Sanskrit word "Chin-Chayane" which means to collect. This collection refers to food. Kaaya mainly helps in food digestion and metabolism. So it is considered as Kaaya Chikitsa that means treatment of disease due to metabolism problem in body. Imbalance of kaaya may occurs which result in many diseases. It deals with treatment of general diseases like fever, cold, cough and many others by balancing agni in body. Treatment may be internal or external.

Internal Treatment

The medicines are given orally or through Sodhana i.e. eliminative procedures of Panchakarma means five treatments which are Vamana (Emesis), Virechana (purgation), Basti (Enema), Nasya (Nasal medications) and Raktamokshna (Blood-letting).

External Treatment

It involves local application of creams (lepan), lotions and ointments.

Baala Chikitsa

It is also called Kaumara Bhritya. Baala Chikitsa is the branch of Ayurveda which is concerned with treatment of children. In this the care of baby and mother is discussed. This branch deals with child care and it includes diseases of children, causes of vitiation of breast milk, diseases caused by this vitiated milk and their treatment, any infection in child. It also includes methods of conception, age, gender, childhood diseases.

To Treat Children Three Things must be Remembered:-

- Children cannot explain their problem.
- Dose regimen is different for children.
- Medicines must be palatable.

According to Acharya Harita, antenatal care and management of puerperium (end stage of pregnancy) is also included in this branch.

Graha Chikitsa

It is the branch of ayurvedic science which deals with treatment of diseases of mind. Management of psychiatric disease like Unmada and Apasmara are also under this branch. Besides herbs, diet chart, yoga therapy, deep-breathing and mantra chikitsa etc are used.

Urdhyaanga Chikitsa

It is also called Shalakaya Tantra. The Physician uses a special instrument called Shalaka. It mainly deals with treatment of upper part of body that are eyes, nose, throat and ears.

Shalyaroga Chikitsa

Shalya means foreign, roga means disease. It is also mentioned in Susruta samhita which is synonym for surgery. This branch deals with surgical procedures. This is done with various instruments like scissors, scalpel etc. Various operations like cataract, kidney stones, piles or even perforations of abdomen were described by Sushrutacharya. Sushruta is considered as father of Plastic Surgery.

Damstra Chikitsa

This branch deals with study and treatment of toxins or poisons like air and water pollution, toxins in animals, minerals and vegetables.

Jara Chikitsa

Jara means old age. It is also known as Rasayana means rejuvenating property. It deals with various diseases associated with aging process. Its main aim is to achieve long and healthy life. It includes different aspects like longevity, memory, complexion, glow, strength of senses.

Vajjikaran Chikitsa

(Vaji - Horse) As per Ayurveda, sex is one of the important aspect of life this branch deals with pleasure and satisfaction of sex. It also deals with the diseased conditions related to infertility problem and problems with shukra dhatus or vital reproductive fluid in the body.

SIGNIFICANCE OF AYURVEDIC MEDICINAL PLANTS

Traditional Indian medicine (ayurveda) is becoming increasingly popular, with many chronic conditions responding to it well. Most patients begin to take conventional medications as soon as their diagnoses are made, so ayurvedic treatments are usually undergone alongside and/or after conventional medical approaches. A detailed knowledge of the action of food, spices, and medicinal plants is needed in order to understand their potential influence fully. While societal use of ayurvedic plants and Indian spices is commonplace, without ill effect, the use of more concentrated products made from single plants, often in the form of teas or tablets, is of more concern. The mechanisms by which polyherbal drugs and their extracts act differ in many respects from the actions of single substances or synthetic drugs. Despite the fact that ayurvedic medicines are based on natural herbal materials, their safety depends on their method of administration, taking into account individual's needs and their specific disease conditions.

Ayurveda first seeks to diagnose patients' conditions before treating them with internal preparations, diet, and habit restrictions. Plant-based preparations play a major role in the ayurvedic healing process. In broad terms, there is no substance in the world that cannot be used as a potential medicine. Traditional ayurvedic texts warn against the use of substances that are not adequately understood. Any plant, animal, or mineral substance can be incorporated into the ayurvedic pharmacopeia, but only if it is understood fully, in terms of its nomenclature, identity, properties, and applications. The texts also warn against the abuse of well-known medicines, emphasizing the point that even poisons can have medicinal properties when used appropriately, whereas the best of medicines can be harmful if improperly used. Of nearly 10 000 plants used for medicinal purposes in the Indian subcontinent, only 1200 to 1500 have been incorporated into the official ayurvedic pharmacopeia in more than 3000 years. All plants must be studied thoroughly before becoming part of the ayurvedic pharmacopeia.

Approximately 90% of ayurvedic preparations are plant based. Ayurvedic plants have a stronger action on the body than either food or spices. Such actions enable the plant to reverse pathophysiological processes and stabilize the doshas. For this reason, one should use such plants with caution. Classical ayurvedic preparations, made from such plants, are known as "yoga" in Sanskrit. Yogas have developed following years' of practical experience combining plants to get the optimal effect.

Polyherbal combinations have also proven lastingly effective than single herbs. In ayurveda, most of the classical preparations are polyherbal, with a combination of 3 to 30 plants involved. These constituents are combined accurately, in such a way that the formula is balanced and reproducible. One or two of the plants in these combinations will be active and the others will play a supporting role. The supporting herbs will each have different actions, acting as catalysts to help proper absorption, transportation, and to reduce toxicity. If an ideal combination is delivered, then the result can be excellent, but such outcomes are based on thorough plant knowledge.

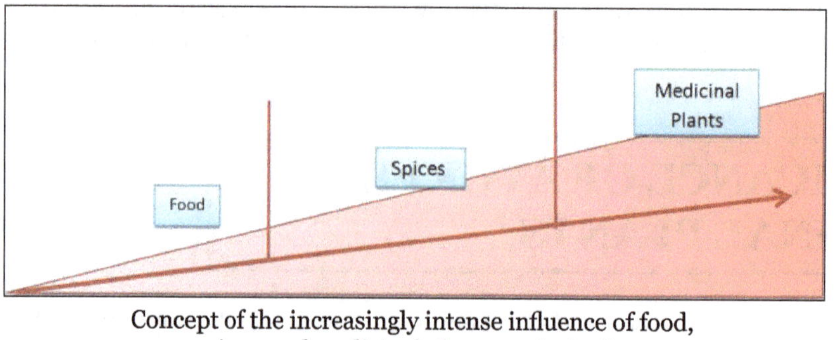

Concept of the increasingly intense influence of food, spices, and medicinal plants on the body.

Ayurvedic Plants: Misuse and Self-medication

While societal use of ayurvedic plants and Indian spices is commonplace, without ill effect, the use of more concentrated products made from single plants, often in the form of teas or tablets, is of more concern. Ayurvedic plants are generally seen as safe and free from side effects, which is not always true. Some of the common plants sold in the market are tulsi, guduchi , and pippali

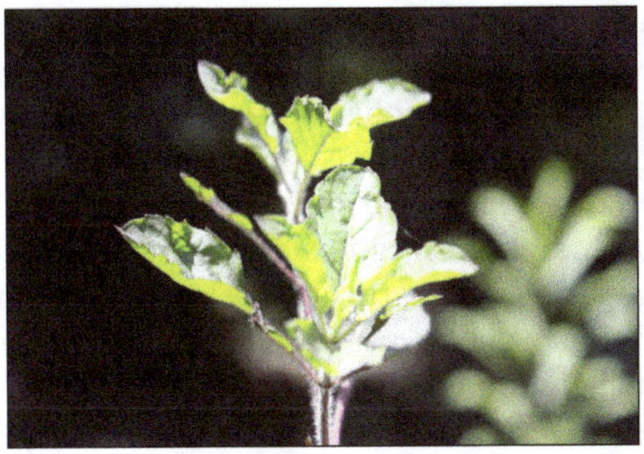

Tulsi (Ocimum sanctum).

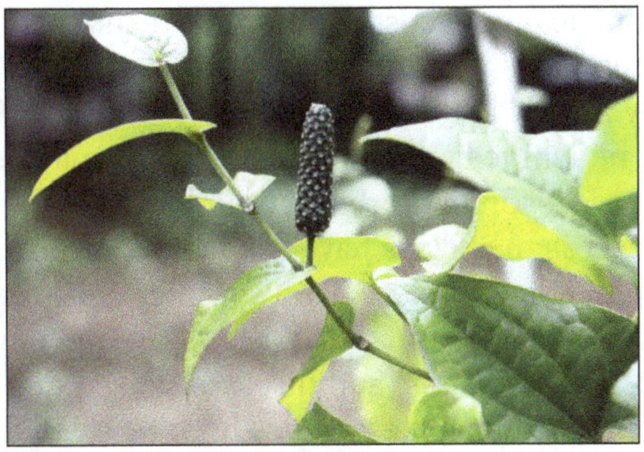

Pippali (Piper longum).

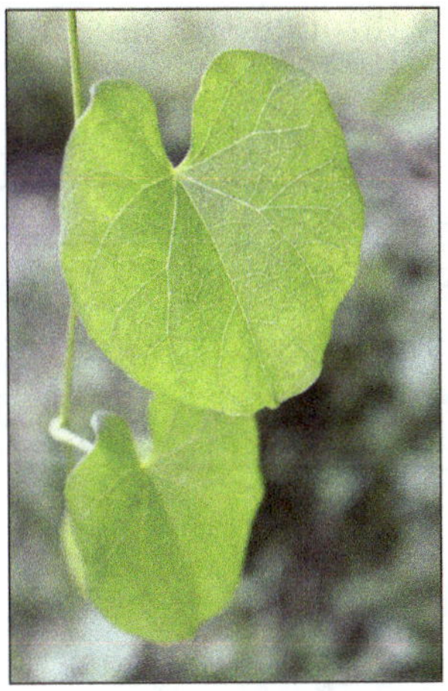

Guduchi or amrut (Tinospora cordifolia).

Ayurveda Branding as Teas

Classified as vata, pitta, or kapha teas, these products are marketed for their supposed beneficial effects on individuals' corresponding dosha problems. From an ayurvedic perspective, diseases certainly seem to arise from the improper function of these 3 doshas. Ancient texts list 80 vata diseases, 40 pitta diseases, and 20 kapha diseases. The more recent recognition of new diseases should make this number even higher. The complex pathophysiology of modern disease means that the symptoms that individuals experience are always a combination of 2 or 3 doshas. This complexity means that ayurvedic preparations must be equally complex. In the classics, 63 major combinations of doshas have been listed and this complexity needs to be considered to elicit therapeutic effects. For example, migraine, low back pain, or arthritis of the knee can occur from vata imbalance. These diseases have different pathophysiological mechanisms, manifesting themselves in different body regions. To treat these conditions, drugs that act on the selected region are chosen. Compounds made from groups of plants are then combined in prescribed ways to achieve the desired effects. This means that undifferentiated concepts of vata, pitta, and kapha-related teas are nonsensical. Most of the above-mentioned teas contain a variety of nonspecific, commonly used, spices. While these teas can certainly be consumed for refreshment purposes, they will not cure disease.

The Rationale for Ayurvedic Formulations and Actions

Ayurvedic products are mainly composed of herbal combinations, ayurvedic formulations also contain heavy metals. Traditional texts such as Charaka Samhitha, Susrutha Samhitha, and Ashtanga Samgraha do not describe the use of heavy metals—clearly this is a later development. Heavy metals are toxic and are not permitted at any level in modern pharmaceuticals. By contrast, in ayurvedic preparations, metals may be added for their perceived therapeutic effects to form rasausadhies (herbo-bio-mineral metallic preparations). In ayurveda, the use of metals and minerals as medicines have been recommended only after purification (shodhana) and that with recommended low dose, with specific vehicle (anupana), for a particular period and obeying dos and donts in relation to diet, activities, and environment. Ayurveda has also described the toxic effect, complications, and diseases caused due to ingestion of raw or improperly processed metallic preparations. Researches have revealed the metal content in a number of ayurvedic rasausadhies and toxicity cases due to ayurvedic herbal consumptions have been reported throughout the last decade, especially those sold through the Internet. Such metals are not found in pure herbal ayurvedic preparations.

Traditional ayurvedic texts note that quality-assured ayurvedic compounds are strong and potent enough to combat disease. The parts of the plants chosen for use are also important. Depending on the plants concerned, and the medical combinations involved, the leaves, flowers, seeds, bark, roots, or skin of the plant may be chosen. The particular combination chosen results from extensive practical experience of the constituents needed to achieve the maximal effect. The mechanisms by which polyherbal drugs and their extracts act differ in many respects from the actions of single substances or synthetic drugs.

Polyherbalism has its roots in the earliest texts of ayurveda like Caraka Samhita, Susrutha Samhitha, Ashtanga Hrudaya, which systematizes the pharmaceutical procedures. The traditional Ayurvedic text Sarangdhar Samhita, which dates from 1300 AD, highlights the concept of polyherbalism in this ancient medical system. Most ayurvedic formulations are polyherbal.While the active phytochemical constituents of individual plants are well established, they are usually present only in minute amounts and are, thus, insufficient to achieve the desired therapeutic effects. Recent research shows that combining plants of varying potency enhances their effect, both when compared to individual plant use and also to the sum of their individual effect. This phenomenon is known as synergy. Some pharmacological actions, from the active constituents of some herbs, have proven to be significant only when potentiated by those of other plants, but are not evident when used alone. Two mechanisms have been proposed for these actions: pharmacokinetic synergy and pharmacodynamic synergy. The former is based on herbs' perceived ability to facilitate the absorption, distribution, metabolism, and elimination of other herbs. The latter concerns the synergistic effect of active constituents with similar therapeutic actions targeting similar receptors or physiological systems. Most diseases are caused by a multiplicity of factors, leading to both visible and invisible symptoms. A combination of herbs may act on multiple targets at the same time to provide thorough relief.

There is a misconception that ayurvedic preparations, being natural, are always safe. This is untrue. Charaka Samhita notes that ayurvedic medicines have adverse effects when prepared and/or used inappropriately. Ayurvedic Pharmacopoeia of India sets standards of drugs/ingredients mentioned in different formulations of Ayurvedic Formulary of India. There are also 56 referral texts described under the Drugs and Cosmetics Act. Apart from these, there have been several other ayurvedic texts written during 1000 BC to 19th century. The numbers of medicinal plants have gradually increased from the Vedic period to modern era inducting more number of indigenous medicinal plants as well as exotic plants. The Charaka Samhita stresses the factors to be considered when selecting formulations' constituents, including plants' habitat, the season in which they grow, the prevailing harvesting conditions, the selected method of storage, and the chosen method of pharmaceutical processing. However, herbs are natural materials, and their constituents may vary due to differing geographical locations, climatic conditions, environmental hazards, harvesting methods, and collection protocols. Such factors make it difficult to standardize or reproduce the quality of the end product.

The concept of bioavailability is broadly defined as the absorption and utilization of a nutrient. The degree and quantity of penetration of a herbal drug, or its active ingredients, is determined by its bioavailability. Bioavailability can depend on the chemical complexity of an herb, due to the synergistic and antagonistic actions of its constituents, in promoting absorption. A drug's hydrophobic properties determine its ability to cross the luminal wall, as do the gut microflora, patients' liver function, and the chemical modifications made by the herbal constituents. Herbal drugs must cross the blood-brain barrier if they are to affect the central nervous system, but there is a dearth of literature on Indian herbs, especially ones with potential antioxidant-stimulating properties. The synergistic interactions of herbs can play an important role in their bioavailability. Long pepper, black pepper, and ginger can all increase the bioavailability of some compounds. Person-to-person variation in gut micro flora and hepatic activity also play a role in systemic absorption.

AYURVEDIC ACUPRESSURE

Ayurvedic acupressure (also known as Marma therapy) is a particular kind of massage or an alternative medical treatment, which integrates the knowledge of ancient Ayurveda and the principles of acupressure, allegedly to completely heal and cure physical, mental, emotional and spiritual illnesses.

According to Charaka Samhitā, an early text on Ayurveda, the cosmos and its correspondence – the human body, are composed of both physical (Visible) and metaphysical (Invisible) forces.

Ayurvedic acupressure talks about 10 elements – 5 physical and 5 metaphysical.

- 5 elements(not exactly elements but like forms of matter exists in our body and environment) or Panch Tatva: – Electricity or flow of charges (not space as it does not exist in our body and environment), Air, Fire, Water and Earth.
- 5 metaphysical elements: – Time, Direction, Mind, Soul and Tam (Origin).

In Ayurveda the pressure points or the meridians are called Marma points. These are considered as energy points, just as Chinese refer them as pressure points, and they help in stimulating not only circulation, but also improve mental and emotional outlook. The Marma points are located throughout the body.

Treatment in Ayurvedic Acupressure can be easily done without needles by:

- Applying pressure with finger,
- Seeds,
- Magnets,
- Colours.

The Acupressure shodh prashikshan evam upchar blakpipol sukh sansthan Allahabad is a non government organization working for the last 20 years in popularizing the Ayurvedic Acupressure

There are many branches of acupressure/acupuncture as we know it today. They are

- Traditional Chinese Medicine (TCM),
- Ayurvedic Acupressure,
- Sujok,
- Reflexology.

These are just some of the forms. The scope and theories of each are a bit different.

Doshas in the Ayurvedic Acupressure

Pitta and Kapha, the doshas. These doshas support the meridians or marma points. But, the therapy restore the imbalance of the ten elements in the human body with the aid of an entirely newly created set of meridians and their points. So, the ten elements are represented on the ten fingers of the two hands and similarly on the ten toes of the two feet.

Hence, Ayurvedic acupressure talks about 10 elements:

- 5 physical elements: Space, Air, Fire, Water, and Earth.
- 5 metaphysical elements: Time, Direction, Mind, Soul and Tam (Origin).

So, there are thirty basic ayurvedic meridians on each finger and toe including thumb and big toe. That makes it 300 basic meridians on the two hands and 300 basic meridians on the two feet, a total of 600 basic meridians. And, each meridian has ten points corresponding to the ten elements, thus giving us 6000 points. Also, the combination of various basic Marma Points develops many secondary meridians. That give us more meridians and points running into thousands. In the Ayurvedic Acupressure, we can see that the treatment is done with the help of 14 main meridians only. Hence, the therapy is quite simple and its intricacies can be picked up in a few months as opposed to many years that it takes to get knowledge of allopathic or other alternate medicines.

Effectivity of Ayurvedic Acupressure

The therapy is effective, and without side effects, has the potential to revolutionize medical treatment around the world. The organization Sansthan spreads the awareness of this therapy. And thanks to this, has extended and its reach to all parts of India and rest of the world for the good of the suffering humanity. Hence, other places have healed through the hands and Ayurvedic massages. As we do in our Ayurveda Retreats, our therapies of Ayurvedic Acupressure harmonize the body's vital energy by working on the Governing and Conception Vessels, the mother, and father of all the meridian pathways. And, it can reach depths within you when an Acupressure point is hold with just the right amount of pressure. This can help you transcend the limitations and traps of negative thoughts and feelings. All this, instead of closing up in judgment, worry, doubt, or expectation, you can begin to relax and open up. Using this therapy balances your hormones. Also, the chakra centers of your brain to bring more harmony and beauty into your life.

Daily Life with Ayurvedic Acupressure

Every human being has the potential to heal and be healed, as Ayurvedic Medicine explains. It can start with something as simple as practice Pranayama, which can clear your head and make you feel renewed and energized. Or maybe it's through a friendly glance or a smile, or the kindness of going out of your way to help someone, as the Karma Yoga. Besides, beyond these everyday gifts, there are many simple healing methods to help ourselves and others get greater wellness. And this is why Ayurvedic Acupressure is so important, you can open your points to feel the healing energy. The acupressure points determinate one of the most powerful ways to do pure energy work, and transform physical and emotional problems.

PANCHAKARMA

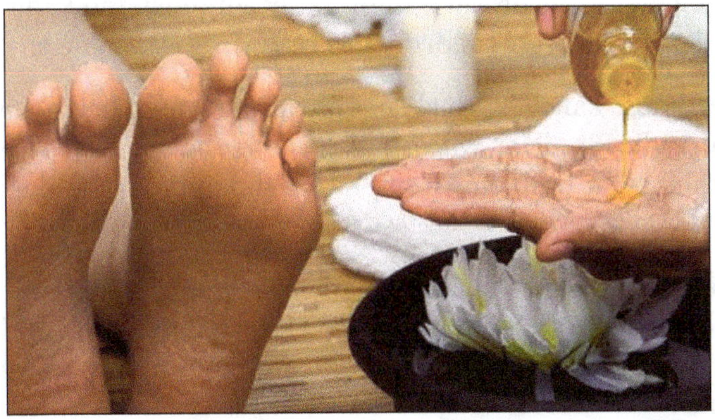

Panchakarma is a process used to clean the body of toxic materials left by disease, poor nutrition and environmental toxins. Normally the body has the innate ability to efficiently process and remove these waste materials, including the vitiated doshas. However, due to one's repeated dietary indiscretions, poor exercise patterns, lifestyle, and genetic predisposition, the digestive enzymes, metabolic co-factors, hormones, and agnis which regulate the body's internal homeostasis become disorganized. This can lead to the accumulation and spread of toxins throughout the physiology resulting in disease. This waste matter is called ama in Ayurveda. Ama is a foul-smelling, sticky, harmful substance that needs to be completely evacuated from the body.

Panchakarma will remove the excess doshas and correct imbalances in them as well as eliminate the harmful ama out of your system through the body's own organs and channels of elimination (colon, sweat glands, lungs, bladder, urinary tract, stomach, intestines, etc). Panchakarma purifies the tissues at a very deep level.

It is a very pleasurable experience that is tailored to individual needs and may involve:

- Daily warm oil massage (abhyanga),
- Herbal steam therapy (swedana),
- Lymphatic massage,
- Herbal enemas (basti),
- Nasal administrations (nasya),
- Other special treatments.

Ayurveda recommends Panchakarma as a seasonal treatment for maintaining mental and physical hygiene and balance.

Panchakarma is a five-fold therapy; it is highly individualized based on the needs of the individual depending on the Ayurvedic constitutional type, doshic imbalances, age, digestive strength, immune status, and many other factors. Depending on each individual's needs, all or only parts of the five therapies are utilized. Specially trained therapists must administer these procedures in an exact sequence for a specified period of time. In addition, although Panchakarma is for the most part a delightful and comfortable therapy, there can be periods of discomfort associated with the profound release of toxins, which does occur. It is therefore essential that a knowledgeable expert who can recognize the signs of properly and improperly administered Panchakarma supervise the therapy. Fortunately these signs were meticulously recorded by the ancient vaidyas.

Like all medical procedures, Panchakarma Therapy always must begin with an initial consultation by a qualified Ayurvedic Physician who can determine the individual's prakriti (constitutional type), the nature of the health problem (if any), and the appropriate degree of intensity of the prescribed therapies.

Panchakarma treatments have been shown to create measurable brain wave coherence and to lower metabolic activity. They allow the body and mind to drop into a profound level of peacefulness. In this state of relaxation, it is possible to cleanse toxins from tissues as well as to release deeply held emotional tensions.

Panchakarma Detoxifies the Body and Mind

If we want to experience optimal health, it is crucial to maintain a strong digestive fire and eliminate toxins from the body. Panchakarma is a time-proven natural therapy that detoxifies and restores the body's inner balance and vitality.

According to ayurveda, good health depends upon our capability to fully metabolize all aspects of life, assimilating that which nourishes and eliminating the rest. When we can't completely digest our food, experiences, and emotions, toxins accumulate in our bodily tissues, creating imbalance and – ultimately – disease. Panchakarma is an elegant cleansing process that releases stored toxins and restores the body's innate healing ability.

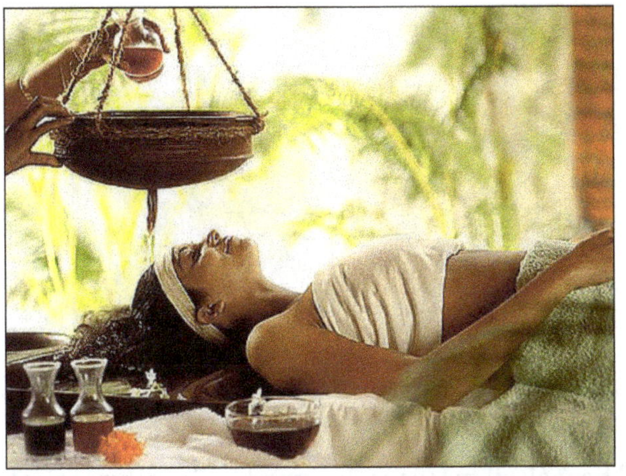

When our digestive energies, known as Agni (fire), are robust, we create healthy tissues, eliminate waste products efficiently, and produce a subtle essence called Ojas. Ojas, which may be envisioned as the innermost sap of our psychophysiology, is the basis for clarity of perception, physical strength, and immunity. On the other hand, if our Agni is weakened, digestion is incomplete and creates toxins that get stored in the body. This toxic residue is known as Ama.

The Foundation for Health and Well-being

When ama accumulates in the body, it blocks the flow of energy, information, and nourishment throughout the system. Ayurveda considers this build-up of toxins the underlying cause of all disease. A common example of this is the accumulation of saturated fat and cholesterol that is beyond the body's capacity to metabolize. Over time, this leads to the blockage of the blood vessels and arteries and, ultimately, to heart attacks.

While it's easy to understand agni and ama in terms of food, it's important to remember that your mind and heart are continually digesting energy and information as well. Right now your mental digestive powers are working right now to break down these ideas into components that your intellect can assimilate. Similarly, your emotional agni is responsible for processing your experiences and feelings, including the smile of a loved one, unexpected criticism at work, or the excitement of a new relationship.

Restoring the Body's Natural Balance

If your emotional agni is strong, you are able to extract whatever is nourishing and eliminate the rest. The inability to metabolize emotions, however, produces just as much toxic residue as undigested food. In fact, pent-up anger, long-held sadness, and lingering guilt are more debilitating for most people than problems with physical digestion.

Panchakarma Treatments

The descriptions that follow cover the variety of therapies that may be performed during a Panchakarma series and represent the actual treatments used in this ancient art of life extension. Two Ayurvedic therapists working in synchronicity perform many of them. Two, three, and sometimes four of these therapies are linked together during the course of one day's treatments.

Abhyanga

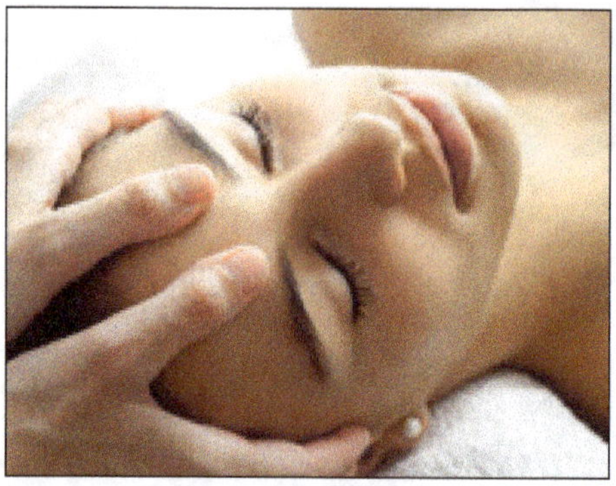

An individually prepared herbal-oil massage designed to deeply penetrate the skin, relax the mind-body, break up impurities, and stimulate both arterial and lymphatic circulation. It enhances the ability of nutrients to reach starved cells and allows for the removal of stagnant waste. The desired result is a heightened state of awareness that will direct the internal healing system of the body.

Shirodhara

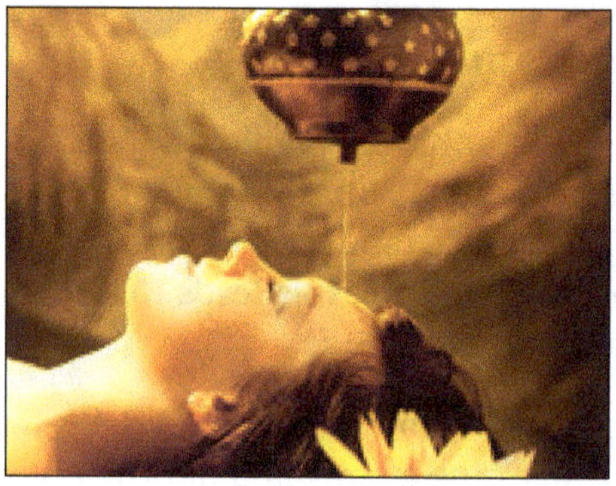

A warm, gentle and methodic pouring of herbalized oil over the forehead, synchronizing brain waves and profoundly coordinating and calming the mind, body, and spirit.

Garshana

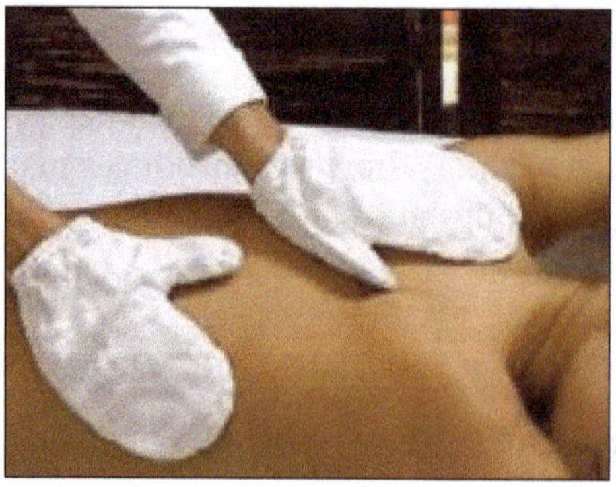

A dry lymphatic skin brushing with either a wool or silk glove. This enhances circulation and cleanses the skin so that subsequent oil and herbal treatments can penetrate deeply into freshly cleansed pores.

Swedana

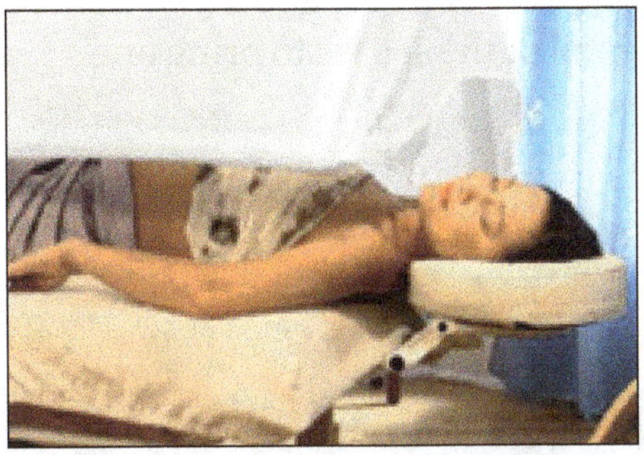

An herbalized steam bath, during which the head and the heart are kept cool (an important difference in Ayurvedic steam treatments) while the body is heated to remove mental, emotional and physical toxins lodged deeply within the tissues. The cool head and heart provide a sense of calm and openness while the therapeutic steam over the entire body can penetrate and cleanse deeply, without overheating and causing stress to the body.

Udvartana

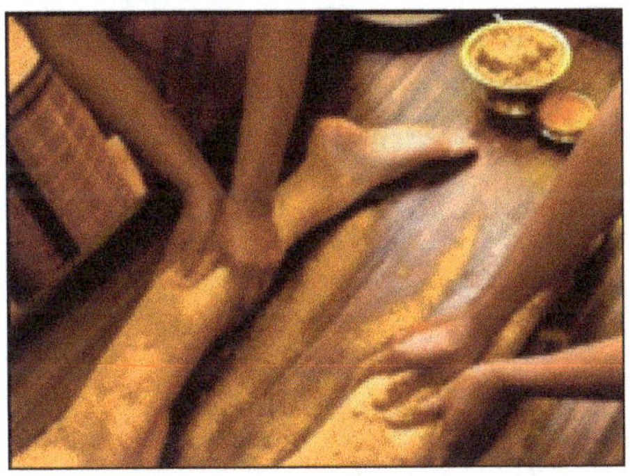

A deeply penetrating herbal paste lymphatic massage. This powerful exfoliating treatment will magically restore your natural radiance. It conditions the skin while releasing stagnant lymphatic toxins from the body.

Five Senses Therapy

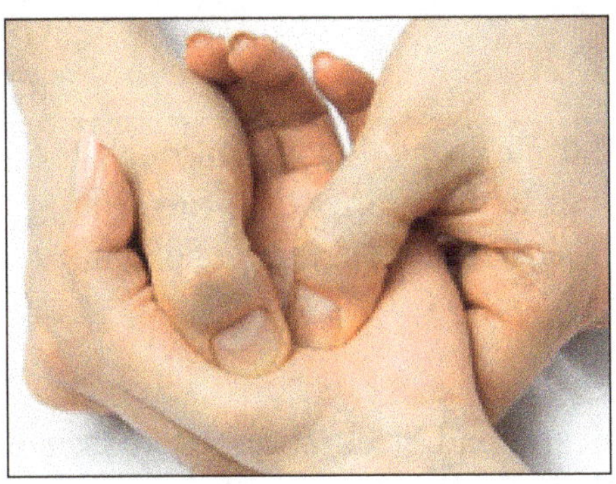

This treatment combines the therapeutic effect of all five senses working in harmony. Sound therapies are specific Vedic hymns and mantras recommended for each imbalance. Touch therapy enlivens specific vital points on the body called marma points. Taste therapy uses certain herbal medicines. Sight uses Ayurvedic color therapy, and smell is accessed with combinations of rare aromatics. The effect harmonizes all of the senses to bring one's awareness to the source of thought and feeling within the heart.

Basti

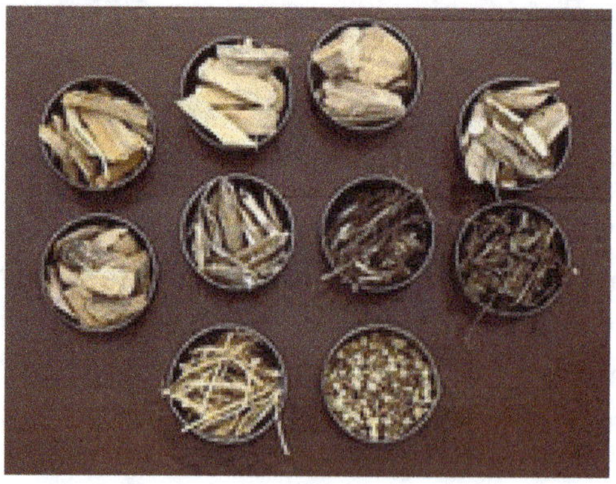

An herbal enema specially prepared to pull toxins out of the colon. This is the final stage of each daily Panchakarma treatment. The freshly loosened impurities from each day of treatment are flushed out of the body via the effects of the basti. The basti also transports Ayurvedic medicines into the blood and tissues in order to transform the memory of damaged and toxic cells. It is considered one of the most important and most powerful aspects of the Panchakarma treatment.

Nasya

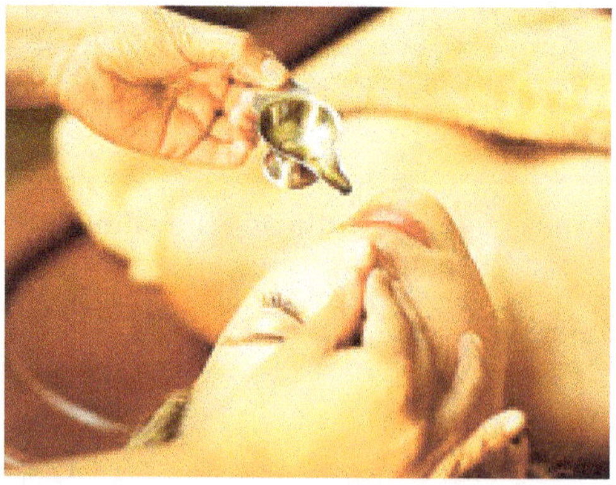

Individually prescribed herbs and oil drops, inhaled through the nose, which clear the sinuses of excessive mucus. It is also an important therapy when medicating the central nervous system. This treatment combats the deep dryness that exists at the root of many respiratory and allergic conditions.

Shiro-abhyanga-nasya

A luxurious combination of a deep head/neck/shoulder massage and facial lymphatic massage, followed by deep inhalation of therapeutic aromatic steam, and a nasal and sinus nasya with herbalized nose drops. This popular treatment is an invaluable tool to balancing most head, neck and respiratory disorders.

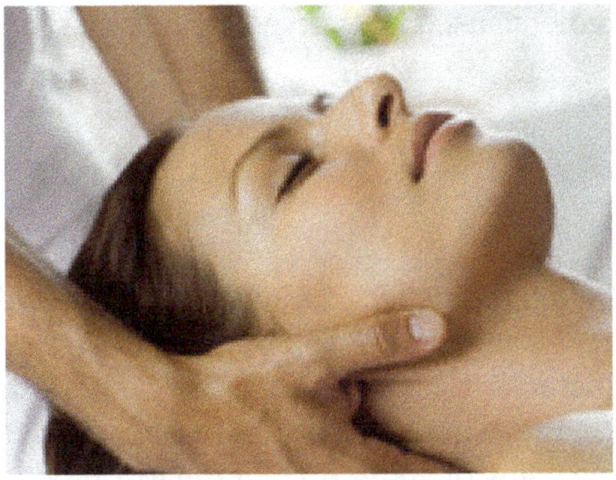

Pinda Swedana

A deep cleansing treatment using rice cooked in milk and herbs that is massaged into the tissues and joints. The treatment is deeply relaxing and rejuvenating as well as powerfully detoxifying.

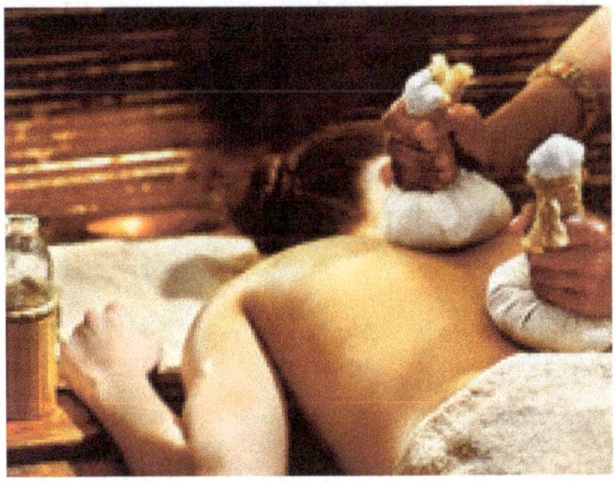

AYURVEDIC CHURNA

Churna is a fine powder made by certain drugs or combination of drugs. Each ingredient is pulverized separately and mixed together. Churna is also called as raj and Kshada. There are many varieties of Churnas and every Churn has its own demand in the Market. Ayurvedic pharmacy comprises of different sections such as Vati, Asava, Arista, Lehya, Lepa etc under one unit.

It is one of the traditional medicinal systems, with an established history of many centuries. It is based on the belief that health and wellness depend on a delicate balance between the mind, body, and spirit.

The primary focus of Ayurvedic medicine is to promote good health and prevent Illness, rather than fight disease. Other traditional systems include Siddha, Unani, Iranian, Islamic, Vietnamese, Chinese, Acupuncture, Muti, Ifá, African and other treatments all over the globe. When adopted outside of its traditional culture, traditional medicine is often called complementary and alternative medicine (CAM)

There are three kinds of ingredients used in Ayurvedic medicines:

- Herbal,
- Mineral,
- Animal.

The herbal medicines dominate the practice of Ayurveda. The worldwide use of herbal products decreased in the 20th century as these were believed to be less profitable than synthetic drugs and medicines. Post 1960, increasing concerns over the side effects of the synthetic drugs and medicines led to an increase in the demand for traditional alternative medicines across the world. Herbal medicine is still the mainstay of about 60% of the world population, mainly in developing countries for their primary healthcare needs.

This potential also needs to be tapped since our country has a lot of medicinal plants, plants with essential oils and the demand in the overseas markets for its concentrates is growing fast. Since the flavourists and perfume experts are facing the challenging tasks of creating and developing complex compositions to meet the present and future consumer demand, it is also necessary to set up world standard research and development facilities in this sector.

The proposed manufacturing facility for Ayurveda Churna would be a GMP certified facility, licensed by the State Drug controlling authority. The facility will focus on "new generation medicines" instead of classical Ayurvedic products.

DINACHARYA

Ayurveda is all about balance. A healthy mind leads to a healthy body; what you think affects how you physically feel; what you eat and drink has an effect on your mind. Ayurveda in daily life is based on Dinacharya, In order to keep your doshas (biological energies of the body and mind) balanced, and your agni (digestion and metabolism) in proper order, each individual is prescribed a daily routine aligned with nature's cycles. When followed correctly, it will enable you to make the most of your life by strengthening immunity and purifying the body of wastes.

Here are 11 ways to introduce Ayurveda into your daily life:

Arising

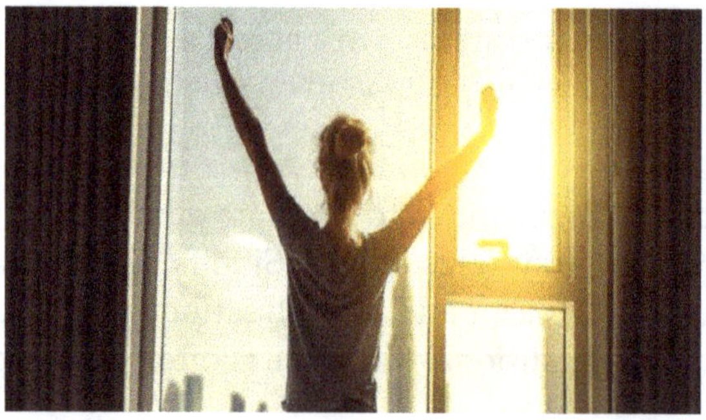

Since our bodies are naturally tuned-in to the rising and setting of the sun, the ideal time to wake up is at dawn. This allows the cells in your system to soak up the tempered rays of the sun and get charged for the day ahead. Drinking a glass of lukewarm water helps to flush out any toxins that may have accumulated in your body overnight.

Natural Urges

The Vata dosha rules the last portion of the night and is involved in the process of elimination. For the body to function properly, sunrise is the best time to get rid of your body's physical waste. Proper elimination also helps to remove Kapha dosha that occurs naturally while you sleep. Defecation is ideal once or twice a day. If you notice any changes that indicate poor digestion during this process, fasting is a good way to correct the imbalance. Try to avoid suppressing any physical urge for elimination as this can lead to discomfort, and in some cases, even disease.

Cleanliness

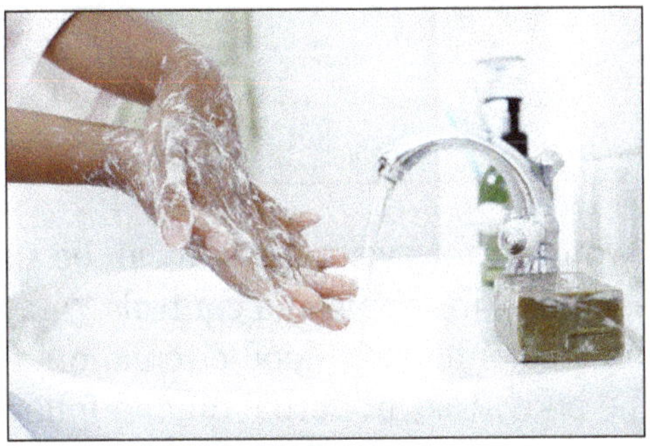

Many diseases and imbalances start with an infection, so thoroughly cleansing your body daily purifies your sense organs and is the first step to living a healthy life. Brush your teeth after every meal, and clean your tongue — it is a breeding ground for bacteria. Occasionally, gargle with salt water with a pinch of turmeric to keep your gums, mouth and throat healthy. Saliva is known to be very good for the eyes, so start by holding lukewarm water in your mouth and then washing your eyes with it. Keep your nails and hair well-maintained, and always wear clean clothes. Being clean can make a big difference in how you feel about yourself.

Exercise

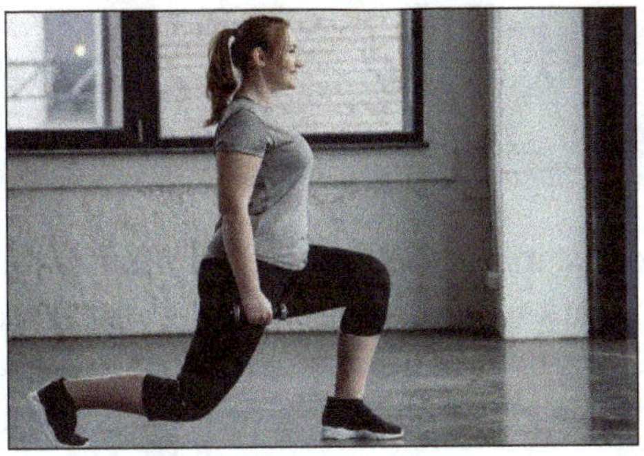

There are two types of exercise: Active and Passive. While both are helpful, it is the combination of the two that will keep you healthy and strong — both mentally and physically.

Active exercises include running, swimming, yoga or just about anything that raises your heart rate and causes you to sweat. Passive exercise is a massage that can help in blood circulation and waste disposal. When done regularly, exercise will reduce anxiety, increase your stamina and allow your body to be more resistant to disease. Exercise depends on age and even body type. Those with a dominant Kapha can handle more intense exercise routines, while Pitta works well with moderate exercise. If you have a dominant Vata, yoga works best for you.

Massage

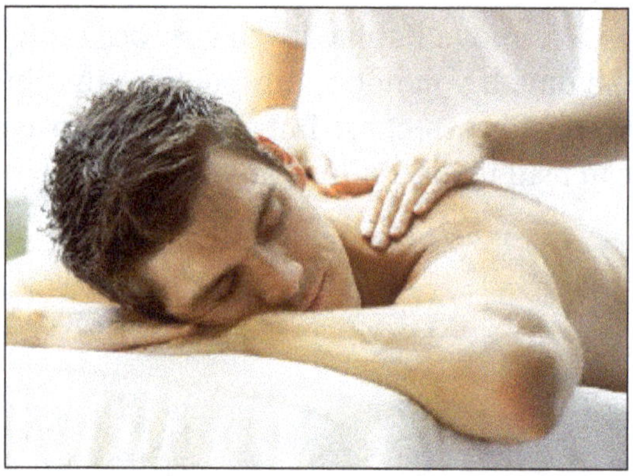

A regular self-massage works wonders for everyone, and can be supplemented with professional attention on occasion. It makes your skin supple and controls Vata by reducing its cold, dry, light, rough and erratic qualities, and also enhances blood circulation, encourages quicker removal of metabolic waste and relaxes the body. Use an herbal oil and follow the direction of your natural hair growth keeping the pressure comfortable. Massage your scalp at least once a week, and if you're pressed for time, just massage the soles of your feet.

Meditation

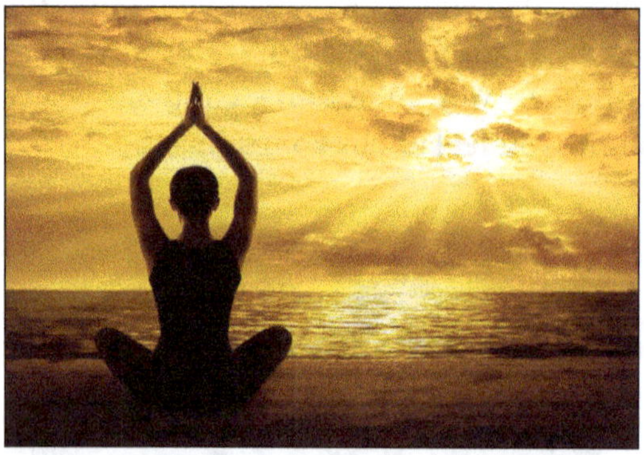

Meditation is ideal to calm and discipline the mind. It eliminates daily stress and strain and works best when done straight after a bath when your body is thoroughly cleansed. Meditation is critical in satisfying the mind's hunger and when done correctly, it can even be nourishing for the body. It helps to control desire and is the key to longevity and immortality. The simplest and healthiest way to meditate involves the sun and its golden color, which is nourishing and productive for your body and mind. This practice acts as the first line of defense against the destabilizing influences of an external environment and will improve the condition of your total health.

Clothing and Perfume

The material you wear should always be light and airy, and as far as possible, made from natural fibers such as cotton, wool, linen or silk. In Ayurvedic philosophy, one should always wear clean clothes and never share, unless it is clothes that belong to a saint.

Energy is brought into the body through the crown of the head and exits through the soles of the feet. This extracts abnormal heat from the body and the polluted energy collects in your footwear. Avoid sharing shoes with other people, as far as possible walk barefoot, and try not to take shoes into your home. Wooden sandals are preferable and a healthier option as opposed to animal skin and rubber.

Using natural scents, essential oils, or perfumes brings freshness, charm, and joy. It gives vitality to the body and improves self-esteem.

Vatas prefer sweet, heavy and acidic scents like basil or amber.

Pittas like cooling, sweet scents like khus, sandalwood or jasmine.

Kaphas prefer spicy, sharp, bitter and warming scents like frankincense or musk.

Employment

Our jobs take up approximately one-third of our lives and success or failure in our work affects self-confidence and self-worth. Keeping this in mind, it is best to match your nature of work with your prakriti as far as possible.

Vata people love work that requires sudden bursts of intense energy. But it also tends to exhaust them. To balance this, they should opt for jobs that give them a routine, and are somewhat repetitive. They need a soothing home and work environment to smooth out their rough edges. They need adequate rest, especially in the afternoon, and should avoid places where the air is exceptionally cool and dry, e.g. temperature-controlled warehouses and mills. Their ideal job will have enough excitement to hold their interest, and sufficient routine to avoid imbalances.

Pitta people are very practical, making good administrators; however, they are not very original in their thinking. By nature, they are aggressive and self-promoting and see most things as a contest that has to be won. Insisting on being in the forefront of all activity, they take on as much work as possible, which demands for their bodies to function perfectly at all times. They do not take delays and obstacles in their plans well, and have to work hard to be fair and keep their professional and private lives separate. They should avoid work that is physically irritating or involves heat, such as welding or metal casting. They should ideally have sufficient challenges to keep them occupied without the stress of severe competition.

Kapha people make great administrators due to their stability and balance. They must make a conscious effort to bring in change and variety to their otherwise routine lives. They should ensure that even though their work might not be physically active, their leisure time should be. They are slow to get going in the morning, and competition is good for them even though they might find it a little stressful.

Choice of Pet

Often an extension of their owner's personality, pets should ideally be chosen so as to have a therapeutic effect on your doshic imbalances.

Vatas get along famously with dogs. A canine's loveable, sloppy open-heartedness is reassuring and stabilizing for their cold, fearful, fickle nature. Some do well with small, furry high-strung animals like guinea pigs that arouse the maternal instincts in the owners.

Pittas are cat people. With strongly held opinions on most subjects, the feline presents continuous challenges with its limber movements.

Kaphas prefer birds. The light chirpiness helps to offset some of this dosha's natural heavy weight. For some, large dogs prove beneficial as the canine encourages them to exercise.

Choice of Partner

Ayurvedic wisdom suggests that like types make better mates because of similar mental processes, attitudes and sexual inclinations. Unfortunately, two people of similar dispositions are likely to have the same imbalances too. Choosing the right partner who will stimulate, and inspire you to evolve into a better individual becomes very important.

Sleep

A state of physical inertia with mental relaxation, sleep promotes proper growth of the self. Night is the natural time to sleep and naps during the day should not exceed 15 minutes, except for those who are very young, old, weak, intoxicated, diseased, exhausted or traumatized. Avoid having a big meal just before going to bed.

Sleeping on the right side is the most relaxing. On the left, it is most digestive and increases interest in food, sleep and sex. Sleeping on your back indirectly and on the stomach directly encourages disease. Sleeping with the crown of the head facing east and feet to the west promotes the best meditative sleep.

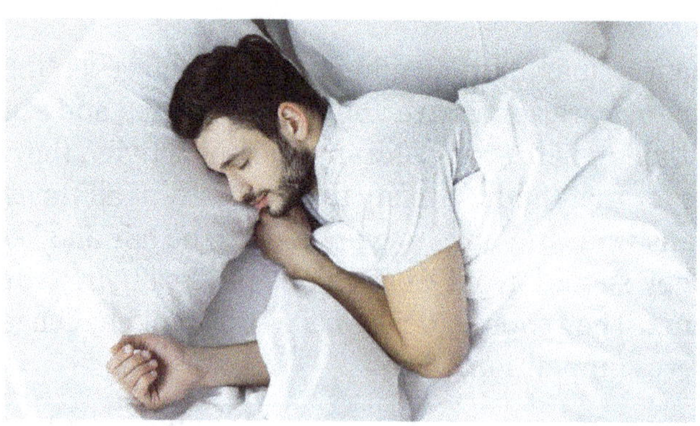

Washing your hands, feet and face just before bed to improve the quality of your sleep. Six to eight hours of sleep per night is essential for the optimal functioning of your body. Practicing yoga is ideal as it leads you into a state of complete physical relaxation with retention of mental alertness and awareness.

RASA SHASTRA

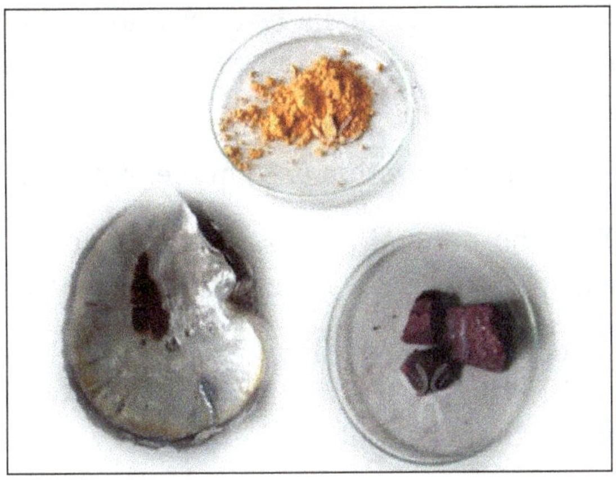

Rasa-Shastra, popularly known as Indian alchemy or Latrochemistry is important subjects of Ayurvedic curriculum. History of Rasa Shastra can be traced to pre-Vedic period, where metals were successfully employed in treatment of various diseases. Ayurveda uses drugs of diverse origins in formulations ranging from herbals to metals. Formulation can be poly-herbal, poly-mineral and herbo-mineral. Rasa Shastra and Dravyaguna are interdisciplinary subjects and they supplement each other. Rasa medicines are widely prescribed by Ayurvedic physicians with amazing results. Use of mercury, copper and gold in treating diseases is documented since times immemorial.

Bhasma of Metals

Ayurvedic theory attributes important therapeutic roles to metals such as mercury and lead. Ayurveda experts estimate that 35% to 40% of the approximately 6000 medicines in the Ayurvedic formulary intentionally contain at least 1 metal. Metal-containing Ayurvedic herbal medicine product are purportedly "detoxified" through multiple heating/cooling cycles and the addition of specific herbs.

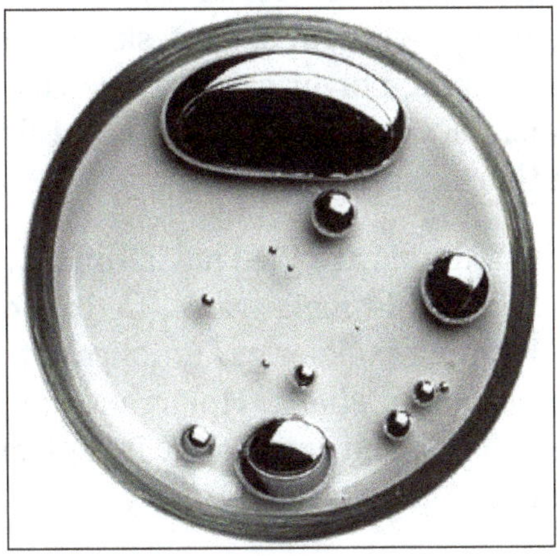

The heavy metals in elemental form are toxic but those in compound form i.e. bhasma are safe for humans. Bhasma are prepared from various metals, metal mixtures and alloys. According to Indian alchemy, bhasma prepared, evaluated and therapeutically used are absolute safe to humans.

Rasa Medicines in Clinical Practice

Aamvatari rasa: Main ingredients are mercury, Zingiber officinale, Picrorrhiza kurroa, Triphala (combination of Terminalia chebula, Terminalia belerica and Emblica officinalis), Cassia fistula (fruit pulp) and Ricinus communis. It is used in the treatment of rheumatism. The formulation is written in Bhavpraksha Nighantu.

Anandbairava rasa: Herbo-mineral preparation used in the treatment of fevers.

Arogyavardhini vati (rasa): Herbo-mineral preparation used in the treatment of liver diseases. Modern investigations have demonstrated the formulation to be hepatoprotective.

Basant maliti rasa: Main ingredients are ash of gold, ash of pearl, cinnabar, Piper nigrum, zinc oxide and expressed juice of Citrus limon. It is given with powder of Piper longum and honey. It is used in the treatment of chronic fevers and tuberculosis.

Chandraprabha vati (Chandraprakash rasayana): Main ingredients are Psoralia corylifolia, Acorus calamus, Cyperus rotundus, Swertia chiryata, Tinospora cordifolia, Cedrus deodara, Curcuma longa, Aconitum heterophyllum, Berberis aristata, Piper longum, Piper nigrum, Zingiber officinale, Cassia acutifolia, potassium bicarbonate, black salt and salt obtained from sea source. It is used in the treatment of urinary diseases, polyuria, calculus, anuria, dysuria, constipation, flatulence, colic, gonorrhoea, pyuria, tumour, enlarged testicles, anemia, jaundice, hernia, lumbago, cough, asthma, dermatitis, skin diseases, haemorrhoids, pruritis, enlarged spleen, fistula-in-ano, menorrhagia, seminal diseases, loss of appetite and debility.

Dhatri lauha: Main ingredients are Piper longum, Piper nigrum, Zingiber officinale, ash of iron and Curcuma longa. It is used in the treatment of peptic ulcer, gastritis and anaemia.

Hinguleshavara rasa: Chief ingredients are Piper longum, cinnabar and Aconitum ferox. It is used in the treatment of fevers. It is given with juice of Zingiber officinale and honey.

Kaishor guggul: Main ingredients are Commiphora mukul, Terminalia chebula (bark), Terminalia belerica (bark), Emblica officinalis, Tinospora cordifolia, Embelia ribes, mercury, Ipomoea turpetheum and sulphur. It is used in the treatment of gout, skin eruptions, skin ulcer, cough, leprosy, gonorrhea, abdominal diseases, anemia, polyuria and dyspepsia. The formulation is given along with Manjisthadi quatha as vehicle. Exposure to sunlight and fire, oil and sour foods and intercourse are contraindicated with this formulation.

Punarnavadi mandoora: Chief ingredients are Boerhavia diffusa, Ipomoea turpetheum, Zingiber officinale, Piper longum, Piper nigrum, Embelai ribes, Cedrus deodara, Plumbago rosea, Inula racemosa, Terminalia chebula, Terminalia belerica, Emblica officinalis, Curcuma longa, Beberis aristata, Baliospermum montanum, Piper chaba, Holarrhnea antidysenterica, Picrorhiza kurroa and Cyperus rotundus, mandoora (rust) and cow-urine. It is given with buttermilk. It is useful in anaemia, jaundice, oedema and haemorrhoids.

Yograja guggul: Main ingredients are Zingiber officinale, Piper nigrum, Piper chaba, Ferula asfoetida, Trachyspermum ammi, Brassica campestris, Cuminum cyminum, Vitex negundo, Holarrhena antidysenterica, Butea monosperma, Embelia ribes, Picrorhiza kurroa, Aconitum heterophyllum, Clerodendron serratum, Hyosyamus niger, Cedrus deodara, Sausurrea lappa, Pluchea indica,

Cyperus rotundus, Rock salt, Elettaria cardamomum, Tribulus terrestris, Terminalia chebula, Terminalia belerica, Coriander sativum, Emblica officinalis, Cinamomum cassia, Vetiver zizionoides, potassium bicarbonate and Commiphora mukul. It is indicated in arthritis, rheumatism, malaria, abdominal pain, dyspepsia and seminal diseases.

SATTVIC DIET

Sattvic diet is a diet based on foods in ayurvedic and yogic literature that contain the quality (guna) sattva. In this system of dietary classification, foods that decrease the energy of the body are considered tamasic, while those that increase the energy of the body are considered rajasic.

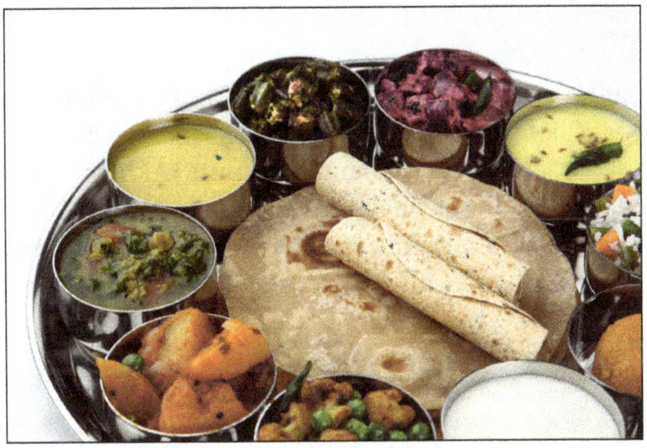

A sattvic diet is meant to include foods and eating habits that are "pure, essential, natural, vital, energy-containing, clean, conscious, true, honest, wise". A sattvic diet can also exemplify the religious principle Ahimsa, the doctrine of non-violence, or not causing harm to other living things, which is one reason that yogis often follow a vegetarian diet.

A sattvic diet is a regimen that places emphasis on seasonal foods, fruits, dairy products, nuts, seeds, oils, ripe vegetables, legumes, whole grains, and non-meat based proteins.

A sattvic diet is sometimes referred to as a yogic diet or yoga diet in modern literature. In ancient and medieval era Yoga literature, the concept discussed is Mitahara, which literally means "moderation in eating".

Ancient Literature

Yoga includes recommendations on eating habits. Both the Śāṇḍilya Upanishad and Svātmārāma, an Indian yogi who lived during the 15th century, C.E. both state that Mitahara (eating in moderation) is an important part of yoga practice. It is one of the Yamas (virtuous self restraints). These texts while discussing yoga diet, however, make no mention of sattvic diet.

In Yoga diet context, the virtue of Mitahara is one where the yogi is aware of the quantity and quality of food and drinks he or she consumes, takes neither too much nor too little, and suits it to one's health condition and needs.

The application of sattva and tamas concepts to food is a later and relatively new extension to the Mitahara virtue in Yoga literature. Verses 1.57 through 1.63 of Hatha Yoga Pradipika suggest that taste cravings should not drive one's eating habits; rather, the best diet is one that is tasty, nutritious and likable, as well as sufficient to meet the needs of one's body. It recommends that one must "eat only when one feels hungry" and "neither overeat nor eat to completely fill the capacity of one's stomach; rather leave a quarter portion empty and fill three quarters with quality food and fresh water". The Hathayoga Pradipika suggests "mitahara" regimen of a yogi avoids foods with excessive amounts of sour, salt, bitterness, oil, spice burn, unripe vegetables, fermented foods or alcohol. The practice of Mitahara, in Hathayoga Pradipika, includes avoiding stale, impure and tamasic foods, and consuming moderate amounts of fresh, vital and sattvic foods.

Sattvic Foods

Nuts, Seeds and Oils

Fresh nuts and seeds that have not been overly roasted and salted are good additions to the sattvic diet in small portions. Choices include almonds (especially when soaked in water overnight and then peeled), hemp seeds, coconuts, pine nuts, walnuts (Akhrot), sesame seeds (til), pumpkin seeds and flax seeds. Red palm oil is considered to be highly sattvic. Oils should be of good quality and cold-pressed. Some choices are olive oil, sesame oil and flax oil. Most oils should only be eaten in their raw state, but some oils like ghee, sesame oil, palm oil, and coconut oil can be used in cooking.

Fruit

Fruits are the major part of the sattvic diet and all fruits are sattvic.

Dairy

Milk must be obtained from an animal that has a spacious outdoor environment, an abundance of pasture to feed on, water to drink, is treated with love and care, and is not pregnant. The milk may only be collected once the mother's calf has its share. Dairy products like yogurt and cheese (paneer) must be made that day, from milk obtained that day. Butter must be fresh daily as well, and raw; but ghee (clarified butter) can be aged forever, and is great for cooking. Freshness is key with dairy. Milk should be freshly milked from a cow. Milk that is not consumed fresh can be refrigerated for one to two weeks in its raw state, but must be brought to a boil before drinking, and drunk while still hot/warm. Pasteurization, homogenization, and the use of GMOs and pesticides are all considered poisonous to humans—as is the consumption of milk from cows that are treated poorly, and consuming cold milk.

Vegetables

Most mild vegetables are considered sattvic. Pungent vegetables like hot peppers, leek, garlic and onion are excluded, as are gas-forming foods such as mushrooms (tamasic, as are all fungi). Some consider tomatoes, peppers, and eggplants as sattvic, but most consider the Allium family (garlic, onion, leeks, shallots), as well as fungus (yeasts, molds, and mushrooms) as not sattvic. Potatoes and rice are considered highly sattvic. The classification of whether something is sattvic or not is defined largely by the different schools of thought, and – even then – individually, depending on the understanding and needs of practitioners. Sometimes the given nature of certain foods can be neutralised by careful preparation. A practice is to drink freshly made vegetable juices for their prana, live enzymes, and easy absorption.

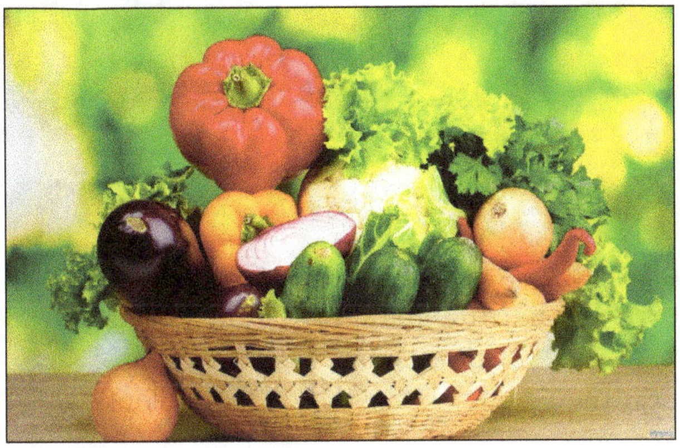

Whole Grains

Whole grains provide nourishment. Some include organic rice, whole wheat, spelt, oatmeal and barley. Sometimes the grains are lightly roasted before cooking to remove some of their heavy quality. Yeasted breads are not recommended, unless toasted. Wheat and other grains can be sprouted before cooking as well. Some preparations are kicharee (brown or white basmati rice cooked with whole or split mung beans, ghee and mild spices), kheer (rice cooked with milk and sweetened), chapatis (non-leavened whole wheat flat bread), porridge (sometimes made very watery and cooked with herbs), and "Bible" bread (sprouted grain bread). Sometimes yogis will fast from grains during special practices.

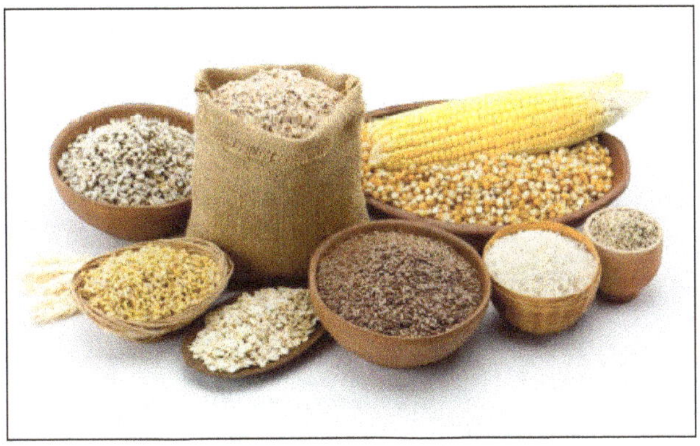

Legumes

Mung beans, lentils, yellow split peas, chickpeas, aduki beans, common beans, organic tofu, and bean sprouts are considered sattvic if well prepared. In general, the smaller the bean, the easier to digest. Preparations include splitting, peeling, grinding, soaking, sprouting, cooking and spicing. Legumes combined with whole grains can offer a complete protein source. Some yogis consider the mung bean to be the only sattvic legume. Convalescent food in ayurvedic diet includes yusha soups made with lentils.

Sweeteners

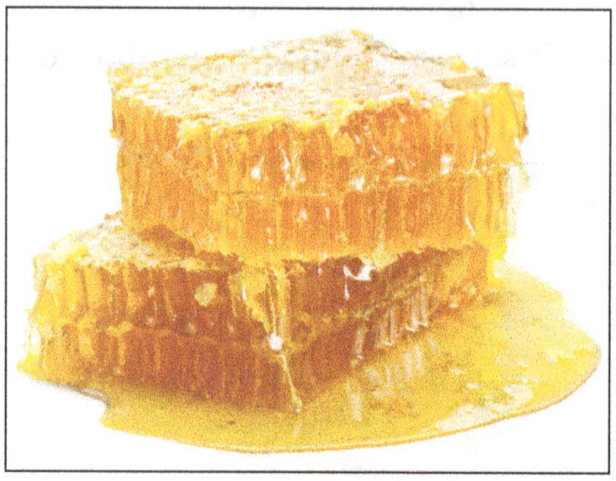
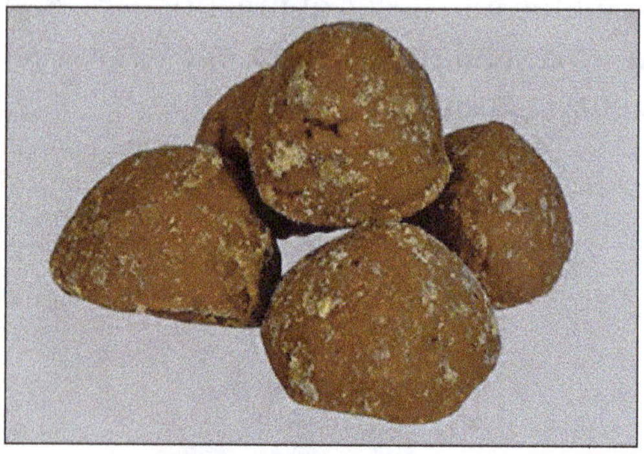

Most yogis use raw honey (often in combination with dairy), jaggery, or raw sugar (not refined). Others use alternative sweeteners, such as stevia or stevia leaf. In some traditions, sugar and/or honey are excluded from the diet, along with all other sweeteners.

Spices

Sattvic spices are herbs/leaves, including basil (Tulsi) and coriander.

All other spices are considered either rajasic or tamasic. However, over time, certain Hindu sects have tried to classify a few spices as Sattvic. It is however considered as inappropriate by purists.

Spices in the new sattvic list may include cardamom (Elaichi in Hindi), cinnamon (Dalchini in Hindi), cumin (Jeera in Hindi), fennel (Sonph in Hindi), fenugreek (Methi in Hindi), fresh ginger (Adrak in Hindi) and turmeric (Haldi in Hindi). Rajasic spices like black pepper (Kaali mirch in Hindi) and red pepper are normally excluded, but are sometimes used in small amounts, both to clear channels blocked by mucus and to counter tamas. Salt is good in strict moderation, but only unrefined salts, like Himalayan salt or unbleached sea salt, not iodized salt.

Sattvic Herbs

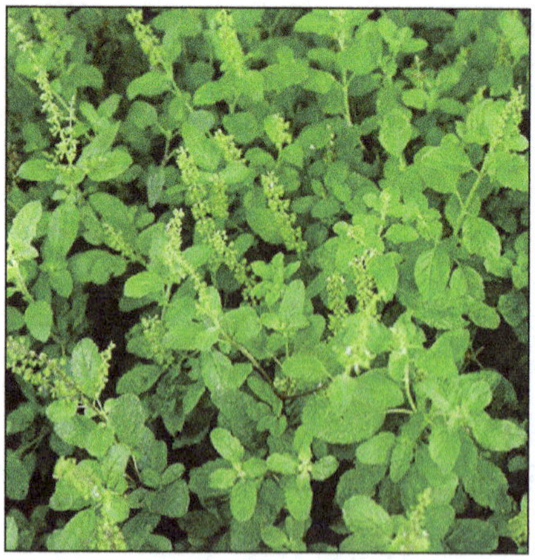

Other herbs are used to directly support sattva in the mind and in meditation. These include ashwagandha, bacopa, calamus, gotu kola, ginkgo, jatamansi, purnarnava, shatavari, saffron, shankhapushpi, tulsi and rose.

Rajasic (Stimulant) Foods

Stimulant foods, also called mutative foods, mutable foods or rajasic foods, are foods that often provoke mental restlessness. They are not completely beneficial, nor are they harmful, to body or mind. Foods that cannot be categorized as either sentient or static are classified in this food group.

These foods are thought by some to cause aggressive and dominating thoughts, especially towards others.

Stimulant foods energize and develop the manipura (navel) chakra and body but do not promote advancement in the higher chakras.

Such foods include: caffeinated drinks such as coffee, tea (both black and green), cola drinks, energy drinks, brown or black chocolate, ginkgo biloba, spicy food, unfertilized eggs, and salt.

Tamasic (Sedative) Foods

Sedative foods, also called static foods, or tamasic foods, are foods whose consumption, according to Yoga, are harmful to either mind or body. Harm to mind includes anything that will lead to a duller, less refined state of consciousness. Bodily harm includes any foods that will cause detrimental stress to any physical organ, directly or indirectly (via any physical imbalance).

They are, however, sometimes necessary during times of great physical stress and pain. They help dull the pain and lower consciousness, allowing the body to repair itself. Such static foods may be deemed necessary in times of war or great distress.

Static foods stimulate and strengthen the lower two chakras, but will not assist in beneficial development of the higher chakras. In fact, they are usually detrimental to the advancement of the higher chakras.

Such foods include: meat, fish, fertilized eggs, onion, garlic, scallion, leek, chive, mushroom, alcoholic beverage, durian (fruit), blue cheese, eggplant (only in Jain customs), opium, and stale food.

Incompatible Foods

Incompatible foods (viruddha) are considered to be a cause of many diseases. In the Charaka Samhita, a list of food combinations considered incompatible in the sattvic system is given. P.V. Sharma states that such incompatibilities may not have influence on a person who is strong, exercises sufficiently, and has a good digestive system.

Examples of combinations that are considered incompatible include:

- Salt or anything containing salt with milk (produces skin diseases).
- Fruit with milk products.
- Fish with milk products (produces toxins).
- Meat with milk products.
- Sour food or sour fruit with milk products.

- Leafy vegetables with milk products.
- Milk pudding or sweet pudding with rice.
- Mustard oil and curcuma.

ABHYANGA

Abhyanga ("oil massage") is a form of Ayurvedic medicine that involves massage of the body with dosha-specific warm herb infused oils. The oil is usually pre-mixed with herbs for specific conditions.

The Abhyanga is a part of the Dinacharya (daily practices) specified by the Brhat Trayi and Laghutrayi series of Ayurvedic textbooks to maintain good health and well-being. Proponents claim Abhyanga aids joint health, nourishes the dhatus (tissues of the body) and brings aggravated doshas back to balance. They further claim it improves the condition of dry, coarse hair and flaky skin.

Abhyanga can be done as part of the steps of panchakarma therapy, especially in the first stage: Purva Karma (pre-treatment), or as its own therapy.

It is often followed by svedana therapy or a warm bath. Abhyanga may be performed by one or more therapists working in sync, but it can also be done by oneself. Oils used can vary depending on the season and the individuals out of balance constitution Vkrtti.

The Abhyanga as prescribed in the Brhtatrayi and Laghutrayi texts is vigorous, and intended to open up the minor Sortas, remove ama (toxins) through the skin, melt kleshma (fat secretions blocking the srotas), and cleanse and moisturize the skin. But Abhyanga can also be used to soothe a Vata imbalance which will bring deep relaxation to the body and a peaceful mind.

- The purpose + Technique of abhyanga.
- The difference between ayurvedic massage (Abhyanga) and regular massage.
- Types of ayurvedic massage.
- The Sarvanga abhyanga (Full body ayurvedic massage).
- Oils for full body massage.
- How to give yourself a whole body abhyanga.
- Finishing up your ayurvedic massage.
- Ayurveda dry massage (Udvartan), an abhyanga variation.
- Ayurvedic massage contraindications.
- Shiro abhyanga: Ayurvedic head massage.
- Pad abhyanga: Ayurvedic foot massage.
- Give yourself a foot massage.

- Marma abhyanga: Vital energy point massage.
- Kerala pad abhyanga: South indian foot massage.
- Sutika abhyanga: Post natal massage.
- Navjat shishu abhyanga: Ayurvedic newborn massage.
- How to do ayurvedic newborn massage.
- When to start newborn massage.
- When to give an infant a massage.
- Benefits of newborn massage.
- Contraindications of newborn massage.

The Purpose + Technique of Abhyanga

Abhyanga is a synchronized massaging of the body towards the direction of the movement of arterial blood.

In practical terms, it means massaging the body in the direction of the body hair.

The scientific reason for this may be due to the increase in blood flow towards the most distal parts of the body.

If the massage is done towards the heart, or in the direction opposite to that of the body hair, the massage may overwhelm the heart through the increased venous return.

Abhyanga may be done using oil, herbal powder, herbal pastes or ghee.

It is a part of the daily routine suggested by Ayurveda. It is used for relief of pain, stiffness, and tiredness.

It also forms an important part of snehana or oleation which is an indispensable prelude to panchakarma treatments, the five Ayurvedic detoxification therapies.

Abhyanga not only prepares the body for panchakarma, but also helps to mobilize the dosha or morbidity from the periphery toward the core in order to get them eliminated through the body orifices.

Vata dosha is particularly pacified by abhyanga. Pitta and Kapha can be pacified with a massage using different massage mediums like ghee and herbal powders respectively.

Abhyanga is considered an important treatment modality for balancing the dosha.

The Difference Between Ayurvedic Massage (Abhyanga) And Regular Massage

Abhyanga and other types of massage are similar in two ways. Both involve basic manipulation techniques that have been developed through experience and have been passed on from generation to generation.

Interestingly, Ayurvedic texts do not give details of the procedures involved in abhyanga but mention certain techniques.

'Samvahan' means gentle rubbing. 'Peedan' means pressing and squeezing. 'Mardan' means pressure massage, which corresponds to modern-day massage techniques.

Various abhyanga techniques have been developed over the centuries.

Abhyanga differs from other massages in that it invariably uses copious amounts of oil for massaging the body.

Unlike massage which is used for recreation and relaxation, abhyanga is a therapeutic procedure used in many health disorders. Medicated oils are used to encourage therapeutic effects on the body.

This type of distinction is not made by modern-day massage therapy unless combined with aromatherapy.

Types of Ayurvedic Massage

Ayurvedic massage can be classified into different types according to the body part involved and the techniques developed and used by different schools of massage.

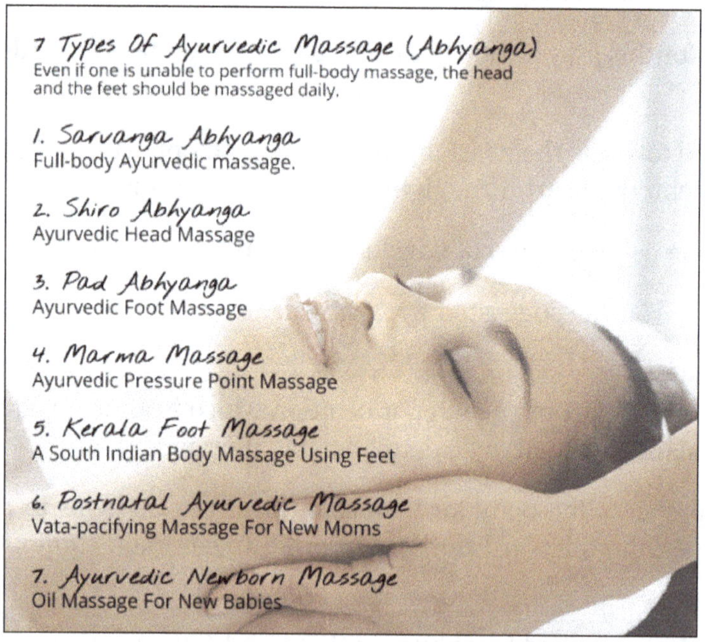

The Ayurvedic text Charaka Samhita specifically mentions the benefits of full-body abhyanga (sarvanga abhyanga), head massage (shiro abhyanga) and foot massage (pad abhyanga) separately.

This shows the relative importance of massage of these particular parts of the body. They can be massaged in isolation or along with full body massage.

To reiterate this fact, Vagbhatta's Ashtanga Hridayam states that even if one is unable to perform a full body massage, feet and head should be massaged regularly.

Other popular abhyanga forms are marma massage and Kerala foot massage. Traditionally in rural India massage of the newborn and post-delivery massage of the mother by the midwife is popular.

Massage is also done by traditional 'bone setters' for sprains, dislocations, and fractures.

Though there are no details of massage procedures in the ancient texts, the techniques of abhyanga have been developed by the traditional practitioners and have been more or less standardized.

The reason seems to be that abhyanga was such a common and indispensable part of the daily routine at the time these texts were written that they did not feel the need to explain the technique in detail.

Only to reiterate their importance, the benefits were highlighted.

Here are the basic techniques and steps involved in these different forms of abhyanga based on the experiences of different Ayurvedic practitioners and abhyanga therapists.

The Sarvanga Abhyanga (Full Body Ayurvedic Massage)

Ideally, full-body Ayurvedic massage should start with the head and end at the feet.

The body should be massaged in sections and not the whole body at a stretch. This is to facilitate the proper flow of blood and lymph and induce relaxation of the body part by part, from the head downwards.

Massage should be done Slowly with Varying Pressures

Firm pressure should be applied on the extremities and light to very light pressure should be applied to the neck, abdomen, heart area, face, eyes, and forehead.

The extremities can be massaged with long strokes in the direction of the body hair. The back of the neck, waist, and sides of the body can also be massaged using long and firm strokes.

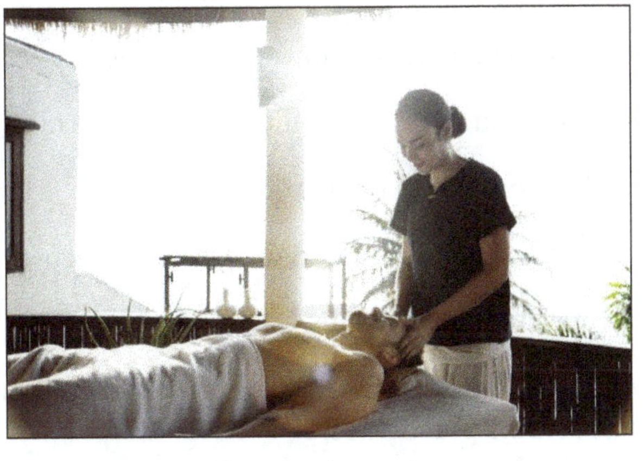

Circular clockwise motion should be used on the joints.

The abdomen should be massaged in a clockwise circular motion in the direction of the large intestine. Move up on the right side then straight across the abdomen and then downwards on the left side.

The massage should be done for 5-15 minutes on a routine basis and on weekends one should give at least 10 -15 minutes to each of the three areas of the body – head, body, and feet.

Rest for 15 minutes after massage then take a warm water bath.

Massage should be done in a comfortably warm, ventilated but draft-free room like a bathroom.

Warm oil should be used for the body and cool to lukewarm oil should be used on the head. In peak summer season cool oil can be used and in cold seasons lukewarm to warm oil should only be used even on the head.

For Pitta dominated people or for those with Pitta aggravation, oil at room temperature can be used.

Oils for Full Body Massage

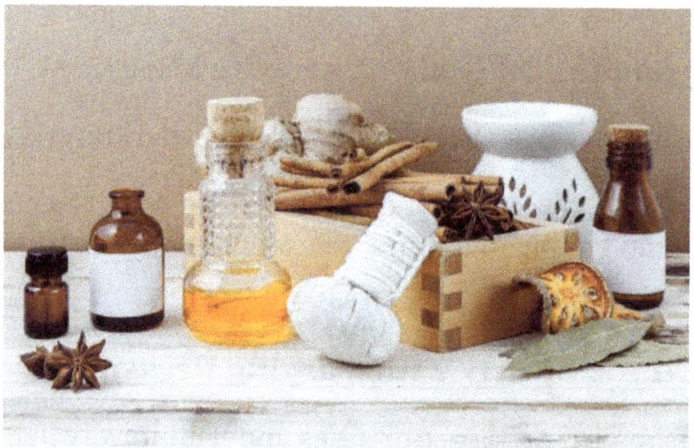

The choice of oils should preferably be made according to your dosha or body type and the area to be massaged. For the head, generally oils with cooling properties are used.

- For Vata constitution, use sesame, olive or castor oil.
- For Pitta constitution, use coconut, sunflower oil or ghee.
- For Kapha constitution, use mustard, sesame, corn or olive oil.

For the body, use sesame, olive, sunflower, mustard or corn oils.

For the head, use coconut oil or sesame oil infused with cooling herbs.

For the feet use any oil appropriate for the dosha. Or use ghee.

In addition, there are several herb-infused oils available for different purposes and can be selected following the advice of an Ayurvedic practitioner.

Be careful about getting oil on your bathroom floor. If your bathroom is carpeted, we suggest that you protect it with an inexpensive floor mat or some disposable covering.

A plastic tablecloth works well. Take a warm shower 20 minutes after your massage. Do not use soap on the body.

Instead, take black gram flour for Vata dominant body types or triphala powder for Kapha and Pitta dominant body types.

Mix these with some water to make a thick paste and apply all over. Rub it off once it starts drying.

It will take away all the oil but still, some oil will be left to nourish the skin.

For taking oil out of the hair an herbal shampoo can be used. Dab the body dry with a towel.

It's best to keep separate towels for massage as ultimately they get oily and need to be changed.

Caution: Never put oily towels in a dryer or hot vehicle as oil and heat can start a fire.

Ayurveda Dry Massage (Udvartan), an Abhyanga Variation

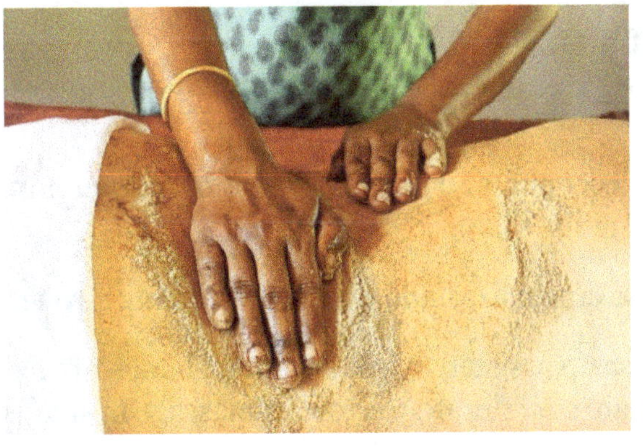

For Kapha types who have a Kapha dominance, and in the case when the weather is too humid, the same steps of massage can be done using raw silk gloves.

Alternatively, first, smear the body with a paste of triphala powder mixed in warm water and let dry. Then rub it off using the same massage strokes.

For the head and face, bare hands have to be used. To enhance the effect, the dry massage can be done in the direction opposite to the body hair.

Abhyanga Contraindications

Ayurvedic massage should not be done in the following conditions according to Ayurveda.

- Fever.
- Indigestion.
- Kapha aggravation.
- In 'ama' conditions which includes an acute swelling.
- Immediately after Ayurvedic detox therapies like vamana (induced vomiting) and virechana (induced purgation).
- In any acute illness (unless permitted by your doctor).

- During menstruation.
- Blood clots (like deep vein thrombosis) or bleeding disorders.
- Hangover.
- In extreme emotional states.
- Dehydration.
- During chemotherapy.

Shiro Abhyanga: Ayurvedic Head Massage

The head should be given an exclusive 15-minute massage at least twice a week.

How to Give yourself a Head Massage

Begin by choosing an oil.

Sesame, mustard, almond, coconut, and olive oils are most commonly used. Coconut oil and sesame oil are best for massaging the scalp.

Step 1: Pour some oil on the crown area and do gentle dabbing strokes with your palm.

Let the oil spread over the scalp assisted by your palms. Then, starting from the sides and working towards the top, give the scalp a moderately vigorous massage in small circular patterns using your palms.

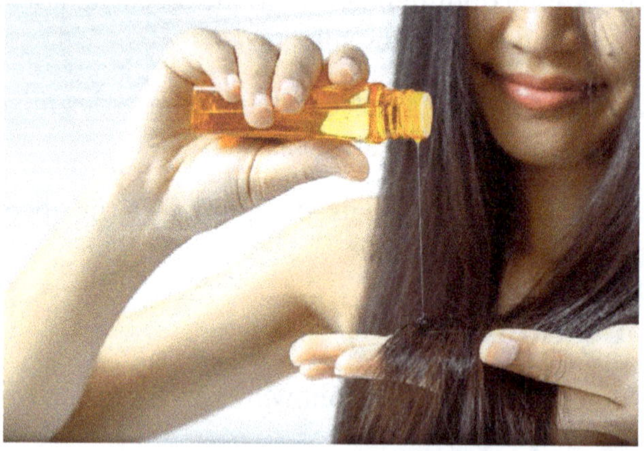

Work your way toward the front and back of the head. Once the whole scalp has been covered, gently massage the whole head in the same circular fashion, with your thumbs and fingers using the flat surfaces.

Step 2: Grasp fistfuls of hair at the roots and tug from side to side, keeping your knuckles very close to the scalp.

Gently squeeze at the temples with the heels of the hands and make slow, wide, circular movements of the head. Bow down your head slightly and massage the back of the neck by squeezing and rolling the muscles.

Begin at the top of the neck and work your way down, first with one hand and then with the other hand.

Step 3: Place the thumb of your left hand under the left occipital area (base of the head) and the thumb of your right hand under the right occipital area. Relax the tight muscles by using friction or a rubbing movement.

Place your right hand on your left shoulder near your neck. Using medium pressure, gently squeeze the shoulder muscle that starts at the base of your neck.

Work your way outwards along your shoulder to your arm and then down as far as your elbow. When you reach your elbow, go back to the base of your neck and do this twice more.

Concentrate on squeezing and releasing the muscles. Repeat on the right side using your left hand.

Step 4: Finally, rub lightly using the flat surface of your fingers and thumbs all over the head; extend this movement to cover your face. If possible, relax for a few minutes afterward.

Take a head bath using an herbal shampoo or an herbal dry shampoo powder. Wrap wet hair and let dry.

Comb hair repeatedly with a wide-toothed comb when fully dry.

Pad Abhyanga: Ayurvedic Foot Massage

The foot massage should be done exclusively for 15 minutes at least once a week or more if time permits.

First Prepare a Foot Bath

Create a foot soak that meets your current needs, using one of the following recipes.

Submerge your feet in the solution and relax for 10 minutes. Remove your feet when done and pat them dry.

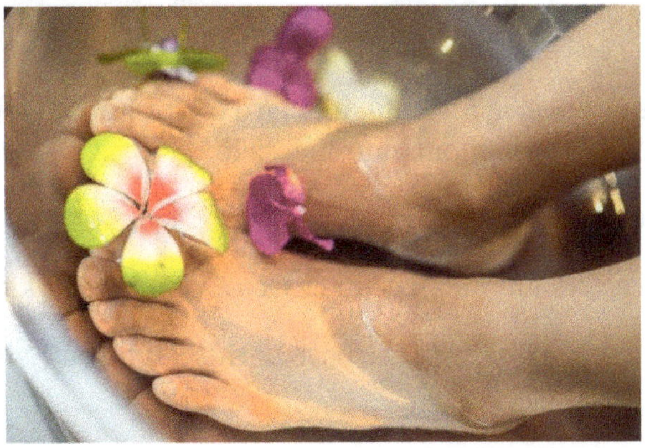

To Cool Down

Pitta constitutions and those experiencing summer will enjoy this cooling recipe.

Fill a foot tub with cool water and mix in a tablespoon of honey and a handful each of dried lavender and fresh rose petals. You can also use lavender essential oil, rose or a Pitta soothing blend.

This will soothe the mind.

To Warm up

Kapha constitutions and those experiencing winter will enjoy this warming recipe.

Fill a foot tub with lukewarm water and add 1 teaspoon of dried ginger powder. This will invigorate the body and increase circulation.

To Relax and Rejuvenate

Those with Vata constitutions and those experiencing rainy season will benefit from this recipe.

Fill a foot tub with very warm water and add 2 tablespoons of rock salt to 3 liters (about 12 cups) of water.

This will reduce any swelling and alleviate fatigue.

Pad Abhyanga: Self Foot Massage

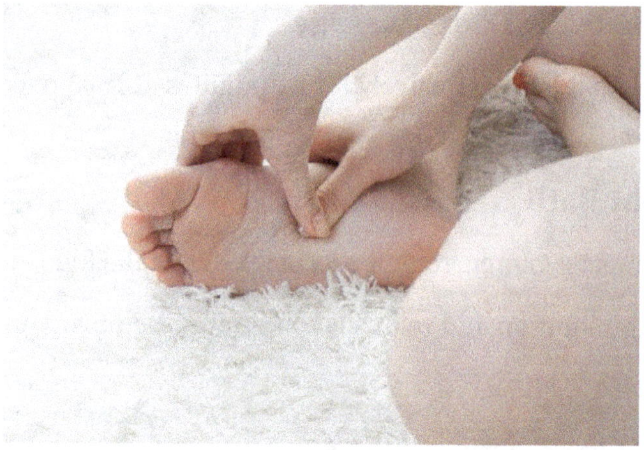

Use slightly warm sesame or olive oil for Vata, mustard oil for Kapha or ghee/coconut oil for Pitta. Apply the oil/ghee generously throughout your massage.

Step 1: Start With Your Left Foot.

Take your left foot and some oil and massage in circles around the ankle.

With your right hand, squeeze down from the base of the calf muscle all the way to the heel bone, 3 times.

Holding the heel, flex and extend the ball of the foot several times.

Massage the spaces between all the toes, pinching the webbing between your index finger and thumb. Glide your thumbs up and down the grooves between the tendons on the top of the foot.

Step 2: Now turn your foot over so the sole is facing you and hold it in both hands, with your thumbs just under the ball of the foot.

Press your fingers into the top side of the foot, stretching the base of the toes apart.

Then use your thumbs to "milk" each toe, sliding from the base over the tip of each toe several times.

Step 3: Next, massage vigorously from heel to toe using the heel of your hand.

Walk your thumbs along the outer edges of the foot, along the arch, and deeply into the edge of the heel. Use your knuckles to massage the arch.

Hold your ankle with your left hand and the top of your foot with the right, rotating the foot clockwise, then counterclockwise.

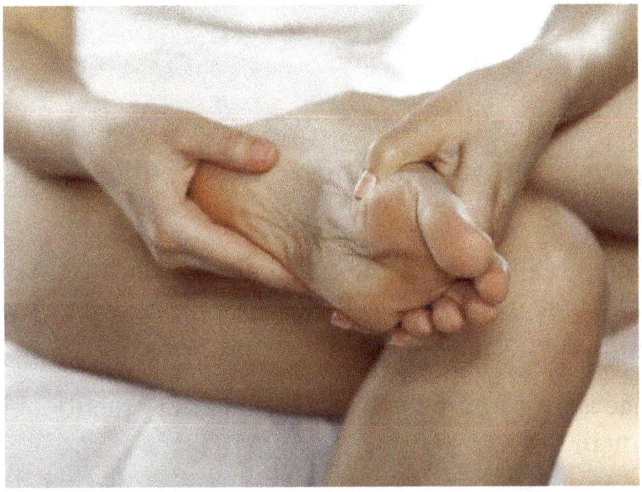

Step 4: Grasp your big toe and rotate it fully, as if you were drawing a large circle with the tip of the toe.

Then rub the toes between the palms of your hands and massage the base of each toe with your thumb.

Finally, using the flat palm of your left hand, massage the entire sole of your foot in a figure pattern.

Step 5: To finish, pat the sole of your foot a few times.

Then press the palm of your hand to the center of the sole of your foot feeling the subtle energy at this marma (pressure point). This encourages a healthy flow of apana vayu, the grounding, and the downward moving subtype of Vata.

Repeat the entire sequence on the right foot.

Finally, rinse your feet with warm water.

Dry them thoroughly and slip into clean cotton socks, which will allow your feet to feel protected, soft, comfortable, and responsive.

Marma Abhyanga: Vital Energy Point Massage

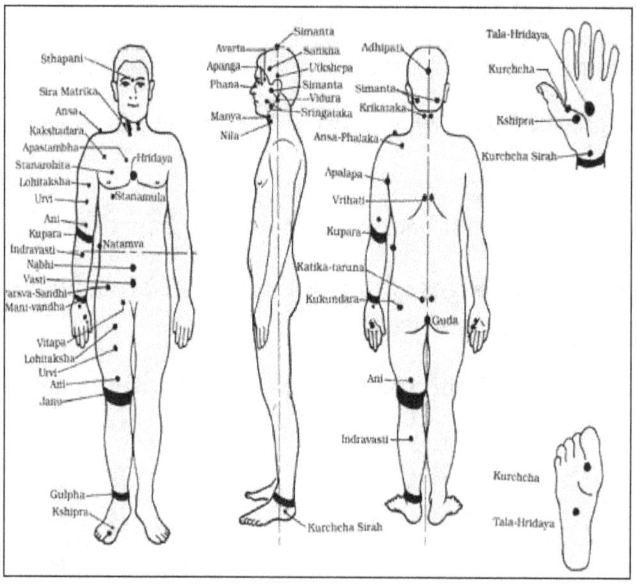

Marma massage is a specialty of Ayurveda. Only a few practitioners are experts in this form of massage.

It involves the manipulation of 107 vital points called marmas located at different anatomical sites on the body. Traditionally they were used to judge the prognosis of the injuries of warriors and were also used to direct the energy flow to heal their injuries.

Currently, this knowledge is held by a very limited number of practitioners in the southern states of Kerala and Tamil Nadu in India.

They claim to manage various disorders related to different organs through Marma massage therapy, relieve pain and improve digestion and metabolism.

If you would like to learn more about abhyanga, check out this Ayurvedic course by Melanie and Robert Sachs below.

Kerala Pad Abhyanga: South Indian Foot Massage

In this unique form of massage, firm pressure is applied by a masseur. He uses his foot while balancing himself on the body of his client.

The client lies on a mat on a hard floor while the masseur balances himself holding ropes that hang from the ceiling.

Obviously, the technique requires the use of the right amount of pressure, balance, and strength.

The body is then massaged from the neck to the toes after applying a suitable oil.

Kerala foot massage is believed to remove pain, stiffness, and edema. It provides suppleness, flexibility, and agility. This technique is traditionally taught by masters that transfer the knowledge to their students.

Sutika Abhyanga: Post Natal Massage

Ayurveda believes that post-delivery there is an aggravation of Vata dosha.

Due to the delivery of the baby, there is a void left behind and Vata finds an opportunity to fill that void.

Unless Vata dosha is pacified, it tends to cause a local aggravation in the uterus which in turn affects the whole body.

To pacify Vata, along with a Vata pacifying, easily digestible diet, massage is performed with an appropriate oil like Dhanwantram oil.

Postnatal massage is usually started the fifth or tenth day after a normal vaginal delivery.

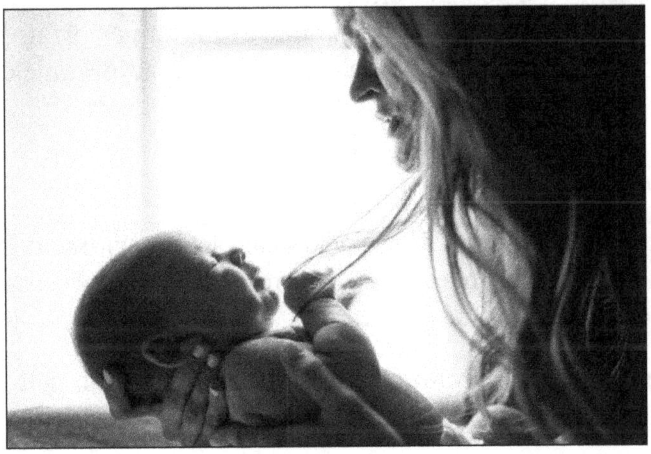

In the case of a cesarean section, postnatal massage is done after at least 21 days.

The basic method of giving the massage is the same as explained above, but the pressure applied is gentler in comparison.

The massage is always done in the morning followed by a warm water bath or warm water bath infused with herbs.

Massage given at this time helps the ligaments and muscles that go lax during the pregnancy to firm up. It prevents sagging of the lower abdomen and prevents various Vata disorders that the mother is prone to at this time.

Navjat Shishu Abhyanga: Ayurvedic Newborn Massage

In a randomized, controlled study on the effects of massage therapy on preterm infants, greater weight gain was reported for the massage therapy group.

The study involved moderate pressure along with flexion and extension of the upper and lower extremities. The massage was given for 10 to 15 minutes, three times a day.

The study reported greater weight gain for those receiving massage therapy versus the standard care control group.

Sesame oil processed with herbs is considered the best oil for newborns. Among the commonly used herbal oils are bala talia, bala lakshadi oil, ashwagandhadi oil, and bala ashwagandhadi Taila.

Otherwise, ghee, coconut oil or just sesame oil may be used. This may be done after doing a patch test on the infant's skin, testing for any allergic reaction.

Dusting Powders for Abhyanga Optional

Dusting is an optional step to abhyanga, but some people find it to be highly beneficial. For vata and kapha individuals, if dusting powder does not irritate your skin, you may enjoy using chickpea flour in the place of soap. Make a paste with the flour and water, gently apply a small amount to the body in the shower, and let it rinse off with the oil.

Dusting powder best accents the positive effects of abhyanga for kapha-types. Vigorously rub an appropriate kapha dusting powder into the body before or after performing abhyanga, either while working in or rinsing off the oil. You can use chickpea flour, but organic calamus powder (vacha) is also nice.

Self-massage

Self-massage, just as its name suggests, is the act of massaging yourself. However, it is important to note that performing abhyanga on yourself is a more involved process than simply slathering some oil on your neck or back for a few minutes.

Ayurveda recommends spending a minimum of fifteen minutes on self-massage each time you practice it, devoting love and attention to each of the tissue layers as you nourish them with a warm Ayurvedic oil.

Benefits of Self-massage

Although receiving a massage from a professional massage therapist is sometimes advised, there is a lot to be gained by learning and practicing Ayurvedic self-massage techniques. With self-massage, the fantastic benefits of abhyanga become readily available to you in the comfort of your own home. Self-massage, over time, becomes a regular act of self-love you can look forward to every day.

Choosing the Right Abhyanga Oil

Ayurveda teaches us that like increases like and that opposites balance, so when it comes to choosing the right oil, your decision should take into account the doshas: vata, pitta, and kapha, and how the qualities of the doshas impact the following:

- Your current state of balance (vikriti): If you currently have a dosha that is high, it is beneficial to follow a dosha-pacifying abhyanga for that dosha. For example, if you are nervous, anxious, and you feel cold and dry, vata is likely to be high in your vikriti and using a vata-pacifying oil for your abhyanga would be most beneficial.
- Your ayurvedic constitution (prakriti): If none of your doshas are currently out of balance, it is good to consider the dominant doshas in your constitution, or prakriti, to maintain balance. For example, if you are feeling healthy and pitta is your dominant dosha, and if

the weather is hot and humid (which tends to aggravate pitta) it would generally be best to choose a pitta-pacifying oil. This brings us to the next factor to keep in mind.

- Your environment: The doshas have an impact on the current season and weather. Fall through early winter is considered vata season, late winter through spring is considered kapha season, and pitta season occurs in the summertime. There are many steps you can take to maintain balance according to the seasons, and selecting a massage oil that will keep you in balance is one of them.

List of Ayurvedic Oils

Because there are so many different ways that the act of massaging with oil can support the body, mind, and spirit, we created an entire organic line of specialized herbal oils you can choose from. Using a plain carrier oil is also an option, but using herbal oils created for specific dosha-balancing intentions are especially good choices for full body self-massage.

Oils for Vata

The primary qualities of vata are dry, light, cool, rough, subtle, and mobile. Most of these qualities are opposite to those of oil, so there are quite a few oils that can help counteract vata's qualities. Plain, untoasted Sesame Oil is considered the traditional abhyanga oil for vata dosha. (Ayurveda considers it to be "the king of oils," in fact.) While it is fine to use an unrefined or refined version of this oil on its own, inherently warming nature makes it the perfect base oil for the following herbal oil blends.

Vata Massage Oil

Vata Massage Oil is an excellent abhyanga oil for vata, especially when the dosha is high or elevated. This oil is particularly grounding and calming. The synergistic blend of nine herbs, such as ashwagandha, bala, and shatavari, come together to offer their strengthening, nourishing, and revitalizing properties, enhancing the vata-pacifying qualities of the organic sesame and olive oils used as its base. This oil is the perfect choice for the fall and winter seasons, when vata is most likely to become imbalanced.

Ashwagandha/Bala Oil

If your goal is to increase strength and stamina, Ashwagandha/Bala Oil may be the best choice for you. Ashwagandha and bala are both known for promoting strong, healthy muscles, and bring out the nourishing qualities of the organic sesame oil at this blend's base. Thanks to its potential to help build healthy muscle mass, this herbal oil is often recommended to support an active lifestyle or to strengthen developing or weakened muscles.

Mahanarayan Oil

Featuring over twenty Ayurvedic herbs, Mahanarayan Oil is traditionally used to support comfortable movement in the joints. If you warm the oil, massage it into the affected joints or muscles, and proceed with your regular abhyanga, it can be fabulously beneficial. Following this with a warm bath with 1/3 cup each baking soda and ginger powder (provided there is no skin irritation) can enhance the effects even further.

Vata Oil Alternatives

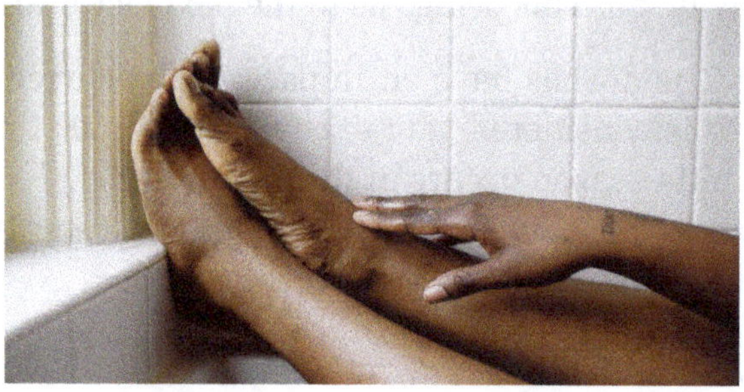

For small, localized areas, ghee is deeply nourishing and hydrating, and it is especially suitable for dry skin. For a formula that adds in herbal support to promote radiant skin and natural beauty, consider using Beauty Balm. This replenishing formula uses ghee as a base, adding in herbal ingredients to support radiant natural beauty. It can be used as a skin cream, eye cream, lip balm, and general moisturizer for the whole body.

Oils for Pitta

The primary qualities of pitta are oily, sharp, hot, light, fleshy-smelling, spreading, and liquid. Traditionally, light, cooling oils have been considered best for balancing pitta, such as Sunflower Oil or Coconut Oil. Cooling effect aside, the addition of herbs can greatly enhance the pitta-pacifying properties of these oils, especially since the concept of oil and the pitta dosha share a number of qualities. The following are some of our favorite herbal oils for keeping the pitta dosha balanced.

Pitta Massage Oil

Pitta Massage Oil is an excellent choice if you have a little more heat in your system and would like to keep pitta balanced or would like cooling support during the summer season. It combines herbs like manjistha, brahmi/gotu kola, shatavari, guduchi, and licorice to cool, soothe, and relax the body and mind.

Bhringaraj Oil

Infused with bhringaraj, known in Ayurveda as the "ruler of hair," Bhringaraj Oil is a great choice for a relaxing scalp massage with added hair benefits.

Brahmi Oil

We offer two varieties of this classic Ayurvedic oil. Also known as gotu kola, brahmi is considered to be one of the best Ayurvedic herbs for the mind. Try Brahmi Oil with Sesame if you want to retain some warmth, or Brahmi Oil with Coconut for maximum coolness.

Neem Oil

For skin that is showing the signs of excess pitta, Neem Oil is an excellent choice. Neem is an intensely cooling herb, which is why our Neem Oil uses a base of warming sesame oil.

Oils for Kapha

The main qualities of kapha are oily, cool, heavy, slow, smooth, soft, and static. Kapha and oil share most qualities. Because like increases like, using oil, especially cool oil, may increase kapha rather than decrease it. However, because oil has the ability to absorb the qualities of substances it is prepared with, appropriate herbal oils can actually decrease kapha. Oil combinations that feature heating, invigorating herbs and a lighter carrier oil are best advised for this dosha.

Kapha Massage Oil

A warming and revitalizing blend, Kapha Massage Oil includes herbs like punarnava, chitrak, calamus, and rosemary. Together, the herbs work together to create an energizing, activating, and mobilizing oil. It is a fantastic choice for the spring season or any time kapha is elevated.

Used with a more vigorous massage, this oil helps to stimulate circulation and lymphatic movement, bringing energy to the body and mind.

Sesame Oil, Almond Oil or Corn Oil

These plain oils are considered warming and therefore good choices for kapha when used with a vigorous, energizing self-massage. If using Sesame Oil, opt for untoasted varieties that have a lighter scent. Our Refined Sesame Oil is an option you might consider.

Tridoshic Massage Oil

Daily Massage Oil is your tridoshic go-to oil for all doshas and can be used anytime, anywhere. It combines powerful Ayurvedic herbs like guduchi to soothe and rejuvenate, bala to strengthen, and arjuna and tulsi to invigorate, promote circulation, and support the lymphatic system. Brahmi/gotu kola and bhringaraj are added to further support and steady the mind.

Why is Massage Recommended in Ayurveda?

The act of massage itself melts away tension and stress from the muscles. Ayurveda believes that these inherent Ayurvedic massage benefits are further enhanced with the addition of an Ayurvedic massage oil. Health benefits from implementing a daily oil rub into your morning or evening routine include:

- Musculoskeletal and nervous system health.
- Proper circulation and lymph drainage.
- Improved sleep patterns.
- Softer, stronger skin.
- Healthy vision.
- Graceful aging.
- Lustrous hair.

- Firm, strong limbs.
- Tone and vigor for the body's tissues.
- Increased longevity.
- Nourishment for the whole body.

In Ayurveda, there is an inherent connection between enveloping the body in oil and enveloping it in love. Both experiences can give a deep feeling of stability, warmth, and comfort. Sneha—oil and love—is sukshma, or "subtle." This allows it to pass through minute channels in the body and penetrate deep layers of tissue (dhatus).

SHIRODHARA

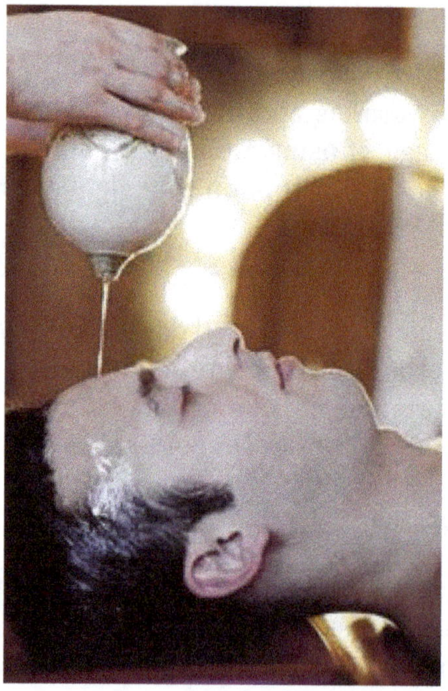

Shirodhara massage is a classic Ayurvedic therapy, which includes pouring of warm herbal oil on the forehead in a continuous stream. Ayurvedic Shirodhara therapy is very effective in promoting sound sleep and reducing stress. Shirodhara treatment is one among the Bahiparimarjana chikitsa, or external treatments told in Ayurveda.

How does Shirodhara Massage Treatment Work

Pouring of warm oils used stimulates and soothes the hypothalamus, thereby regulating the functions of the pituitary gland and inducing sleep. Shirodhara stimulates Marma's or Vital Points in the head and improves circulation. The warm oils used for Shirodhara also cause vasodilatation of all the channels and thereby improve the blood circulation of the brain. Shirodhara also reduces the level of stress hormones such as Adrenaline and Noradrenaline and thus relaxes the mind.

Shirodhara Massage Therapy – Stepwise Procedure

Shirodhara is usually practised in the morning or evening. Depending on the 'Dravya' (medicated or non-medicated liquids), it can be called as Tailadhara, Takradhara, Kashayadhara and Jaladhara. Shirodhara is also included as one among the Murdhataila (four special procedures in Ayurveda for the head).

- Shirodhara massage treatment begins with Abhyangam (Ayurvedic body massage).
- You need to lie down on the massage table with closed eyes and relax your body.
- Shirodhara starts with the pouring of about 2 litres lukewarm oil continuously as a stream on to the forehead in an oscillating manner.
- The time duration of Shirodhara treatment may extend from 30 to 60 minutes depending on the condition of the patient. It is important to make sure that the oil does not enter eyes or ears and is therefore recommended to be performed by an experienced therapist.
- You may also be given a mild head massage before or during Shirodhara. Shirodhara may also include pouring of buttermilk, decoctions or even water.

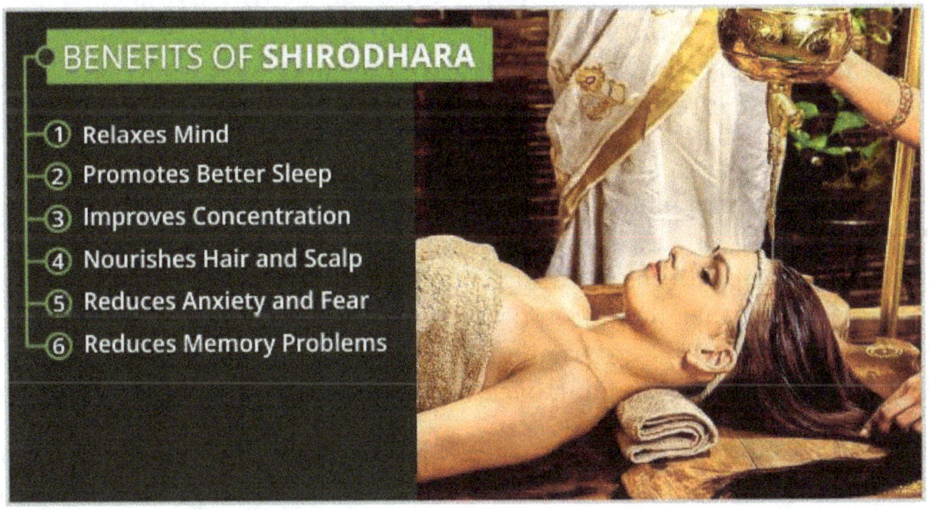

Shirodhara Massage Benefits

The benefits of Shirodhara massage include treatment of Sleep problems, Memory loss, Poor concentration, Chronic headaches, Stress, Depression, Mental tension, Hypertension, Facial Paralysis and Degenerative conditions of the brain. The medicated oils absorbed through the scalp stimulate the hair follicles, and hence Shirodhara is a vital therapy to treat hair problems such as Premature greying of hair or Hair fall.

Can Shirodhara Cause any Side Effects?

Shirodhara is generally a safe methods. However, precaution needs to be taken to prevent the oil from entering into the eyes or nose.

BASTI

As nature transitions seasons and exhibits change, Ayurveda recommends cleansing and rejuvenation to help the body adapt. Of particular focus at this time of the year is balancing vata. There is no system in the body that is not touched by vata, and according to Ayurvedic tradition, vata alone is responsible for more that 55% of the diseases encountered by humans.

Panchakarma is recommended at the change of seasons to help balance the shifts in doshas that can accumulate with the change in environment. The primary treatment in panchakarma that is geared towards vata is basti (Ayurvedic enema). Basti is so highly revered in the panchakarma process that it is said that the benefit received from basti is equal to the cumulative benefit of the other four processes in panchakarma. And that only makes sense, given the prevalence that vitiated vata plays in the disease process.

Basti works in the region of the colon, but its impact is so far reaching and deep that simply calling this process an enema does not do it justice. Recall that as the major seat of vata in the GI tract, the colon is critical in keeping vata balanced in the entire body. In the stages of samprapti (Ayurvedic pathogenesis), vata first accumulates in the colon, and then as it begins to "overflow", it will spread and create imbalanced vata in other susceptible parts of the body. This systemic imbalanced vata can affect almost any system in the body, as vata is a necessary presence throughout the body; it is likely to affect the systems which have some weakness (a khavaigunya). Basti provides herbal cleansing and nourishment directly into the intestines and colon, without having to be digested by the stomach and upper GI tract, as would be the case with anything taken by mouth.

Traditional Ayurvedic teaching reminds us that basti can be used for a variety of reasons, including bowel regularity, joint support, excess vata in digestion causing occasional gas, nervous system support, and healthy sleep patterns. Clearing vata from the system also helps create energy and vitality as well as clarity in the mind. Basti promotes overall well-being, a graceful aging process, luster and a healthy glow. Multiple international studies have been done regarding the benefits of basti, and they also show benefits to joint, back, and bone health.

Basti does have some general situations in which it is contraindicated, including pregnancy, menstruation, diarrhea, inflammation of the anal region or rectal bleeding, and extreme weakness or debility. Generally, basti is well tolerated in appropriate candidates, and a proper basti should result in 1-2 bowel movements with cleansing of the fecal matter as well as a feeling of lightness and a promotion of appetite and agni. If the basti was insufficient, one may be left with pain, incomplete fecal clearing, and/or swelling.

Prior to doing basti, one can prepare by applying warm oil (such as sesame) to the abdomen and lower back in a clockwise direction following the flow of the intestines. If one is so inclined, one can even do a full body massage with warm oil to help with oleation and loosening of toxins. After massage with warm oil, one can place a warm pack, such as a hot water bottle) to the abdomen for a few minutes, allowing the intestines to be primed for the application of basti.

Basti can be classified in a variety of ways. While there are a number of treatments that can be referred to with the term basti, here we are speaking only of rectal basti, as this is the primary treatment for our dosha of choice, vata. Rectal basti is usually one of two major types: niruha basti, which is done with herbal decoctions and is purifying and cleansing in nature; and anuvasana basti, usually done with oil, which is nourishing, strengthening, and oleating in nature.

Niruha basti, which is best done in the morning on an empty stomach, can use an endless variety of hebal decoctions. Often dashamula is used as one of the ingredients, as it is a primary herbal remedy to dispel excess vata. Classical formulas add triphala, rock salt and honey to the dashamula. Modern variations will choose any number of cleansing or rasayana herbs depending on the desired outcome. Guduchi has a cooling, calming effect and can help balance pitta. Punarnava helps balance excess water in the system and can also balance kapha. Other nourishing rejuvenatives can include ashwagandha or shatavari. To help irritation in the system, licorice can provide a soothing nature. And for a cleansing effect, triphala is a solid choice. Niruha basti can be held for 15-20 minutes, or longer if comfortable, up to 48 minutes. Following the administration of niruha basti, one can have a light meal of easily digestible food.

Anuvasana basti is primarily oil based and is meant to be building and nourishing. Locally, providing oleation for any dryness caused by vata can support a healthy, supple colon. More broadly, the oil helps to ground vata and promotes energy and vitality. Anuvasana basti is usually based in sesame oil, which may be plain or herbalized with supportive Ayurvedic herbs. Anuvasana basti can be held for longer periods of time, even up to a full day, as long as it is comfortable for the client, as it continues to provide a supportive effect.

There are a variety of traditional schedules which can use a combination of alternating niruha and anuvasana basti in order to achieve optimal effect. The usual protocol starts with an anuvasana basti to prime the colon, then alternates niruha and anuvasana basti to cleanse and nourish (so the colon does not become overly depleted), and ends with a number of anuvasana bastis in order to replenish and rejuvenate the colon and balance, ground, and nourish vata after the cleansing process. Caraka recommends schedules of yoga basti (8 bastis), kala basti (16 bastis), and karma basti (30 bastis), used based on the degree of vata vitiation. Another alternative can also be to mix the herbal decoction and oil together, blend to make a solution, and administer the basti.

After doing basti, one should take care to follow vata balancing recommendations. Eat light, grounding, warm, oleative food. Rest and avoid vata provoking activity, including excessive talking, extremely windy or cold weather, travel, and busy activity. In this way, basti can be used to keep vata balanced on a routine basis, cleanse vata during seasonal transitions, and manage more extreme vata imbalances that are causing issues in the deeper tissues.

References

- Ayurveda-a-brief-introduction-and-guide, resources: ayurveda.com
- Frawley, david; ranade, subhash; lele, avinash (2003). Ayurveda and marma therapy: energy points in yogic healing. Lotus press. Isbn 9780940985599
- Eight-branches-of-ayurveda: planetayurveda.com, Retrieved 26 July, 2019
- Steven rosen (2011), food for the soul: vegetarianism and yoga traditions, praeger, isbn 978-0-313-39703-5, pages 25-29
- Ayurvedic-acupressure: speakingtree.in, Retrieved 21 May, 2019

- Subramuniya (2003). Merging with śiva: hinduism's contemporary metaphysics. Himalayan academy publications. P. 155. Isbn 978-0-945497-99-8. Retrieved 6 april 2009
- Panchakarma: ayurvedichealing.net
- Ayurvedic-massage-abhyanga: theayurvedaexperience.com, Retrieved 8 January, 2019
- Self-oil-massage, lifestyle, living-ayurveda, ayurvedic-living: banyanbotanicals.com, Retrieved 13 May, 2019

Naturopathy

4 CHAPTER

Naturopathy refers to a form of alternative medicine which aims at creating a healthy and drug-less system of healing based on various medical philosophies. It is used for treating diseases such as asthma and obesity. This chapter discusses in detail the treatment of these diseases through naturopathy.

Definition of Naturopathy

Naturopathy is a system of man building in harmony with the constructive principles of Nature on physical, mental, moral and spiritual planes of living. It has great health promotive, disease preventive and curative as well as restorative potential.

"Naturopathy is a system of treatment which recognizes the existence of the vital curative force within the body." It therefore, advocates aiding human system to remove the cause of disease i.e. toxins by expelling the unwanted and unused matters from human body for curing diseases.

Some Important Treatments of Naturopathy

- Mud pack, mud applications.
- Mud bath, underground mud bath, mud pool bath.
- Hip bath.
- Spinal bath, spinal spray bath.
- Immersion bath, friction bath.
- Foot bath, arm bath.
- Steam bath, sauna bath.
- Sun bath, colour sun bath (Chromo Bath).
- Green leaves sun bath.
- Hot & Cold fomentation.
- Wet sheet pack, chest pack, abdomen pack, trunk pack.
- Knee pack, neck pack, wet girdle pack.

- Enema-warm water, butter milk, tender coconut water etc.
- Circular jet bath.
- Colon irrigation.
- Deluxe hydro massage, jacuzi.
- Hot and cold water douches, effusions.
- Whirlpool bath.
- Under water exercises.
- Magnet therapy.
- Colour therapy.
- Acupuncture.
- Acupressure.
- Reflexology.
- Physiotherapy treatments - Exercise therapy, electro therapy.

FEATURES OF NATUROPATHY

The main features of Naturopathy are as under:

- All diseases, their causes and treatment are one. Except for traumatic and environmental conditions, the cause of all diseases is one i.e. accumulation of morbid matter in the body. The treatment of all diseases is elimination of morbid matter from the body.
- The primary cause of disease is accumulation of morbid matter. Bacteria and virus enter and survive in the body only after the accumulation of morbid matter when a favorable atmosphere for their growth is established in body. Hence, the basic cause of disease is morbid matter and bacteria secondary causes.
- Acute diseases are self-healing efforts of the body. Hence, they are our friends, not the enemy. Chronic diseases are outcome of wrong treatment and suppression of the acute diseases.
- Nature is the greatest healer. The human body itself has the healing power to prevent itself from disease and regain health if unhealthy.
- In nature cure it is not the disease but the entire body of the patient which is caused and is renewed.
- Naturopathy cures patients suffering from chronic ailments are also treated successfully in comparatively less time by Naturopathy.

- In nature cure the suppressed diseases are brought to surface and are removed permanently.
- Naturopathy treats all the aspects like physical, mental, social and spiritual at the same time.
- Naturopathy treats the body as a whole.
- According to Naturopathy, "Food is only the Medicine", no external medications are used.
- Performing prayer according to one's spiritual faith is an important part of treatment.

GRAPE THERAPY

Grape therapy, also known as ampelotherapy, is a form of naturopathic alternative medicine that involves heavy consumption of grapes, including seeds, and parts of the vine, including leaves. Although there is some limited evidence of positive benefits from the use of grape therapy for health purposes, extreme claims, such as its ability to cure cancer, have been widely derided as "quackery".

Grapes have been associated with health for many centuries. They contain organic acids (tartaric, malic, citric, tannic), B group vitamins, vitamins P, PP, and C, calcium, carotene, magnesium salts, phosphorus and potassium, as well as trace elements such as copper, iron, manganese, sulphur and zinc. Proanthocyanidins, first extracted from grape seeds in 1970, and resveratrol, found in grape skins, have been studied for possible uses in the prevention and treatment of cancer and other illnesses, and for anti-ageing. Proanthocyanidins are powerful antioxidants that can block the action of free radicals. Recent research by scientists at UCLA has found that combining resveratrol with benzoyl peroxide may improve that drug's ability to kill the bacteria associated with acne. The presence of resveratrol on the skin of red grapes has prompted some doctors to recommend that adults drink reasonable quantities of red wine to combat heart disease. Resveratrol in red wine is suggested as an explanation for the disputed "French paradox," i.e. the apparent low occurrence of heart disease among the French, even though they eat a high-fat diet. Advocates of grape therapy argue that these antioxidants inhibit the development of cancer, and can be used in treating a variety of other medical conditions such as arthritis and diabetes.

Grapes are said to be beneficial for protecting against cardiovascular disease and, because of their potassium and glucose content, they are argued to be useful for treatment of heart disease by strengthening muscle tone, improving heart function and having a positive impact on convalescence. Alternative medicine practitioners have at times also recommended grapes and parts of the vine for high blood pressure, menopause, varicose veins, high cholesterol, skin rashes, and urination problems. The grape diet was promoted in the past as a treatment to flush toxins from the body. The grape cure is also prescribed for a decline in nutrition, especially with patients with early stage of tuberculosis, for diseases of the liver, kidneys and lungs and for gout and secondary anaemia and, in addition, for mental disease, nervous disorders, and sexual problems.

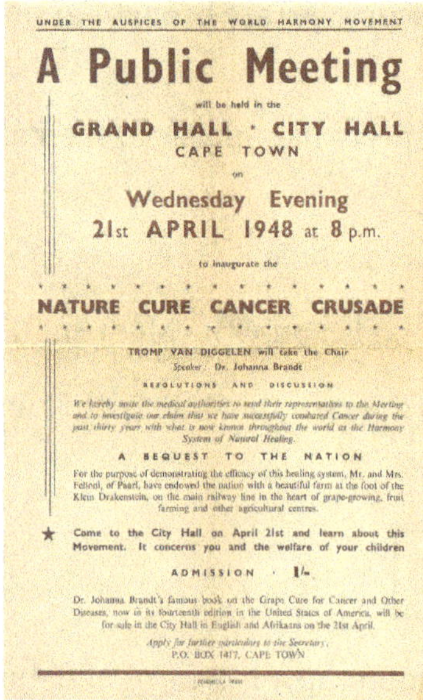

UNDER THE AUSPICES OF THE WORLD HARMONY MOVEMENT

A Public Meeting

will be held in the

GRAND HALL · CITY HALL

CAPE TOWN

on

Wednesday Evening

21st APRIL 1948 at 8 p.m.

to inaugurate the

NATURE CURE CANCER CRUSADE

TROMP VAN DIGGELEN will take the Chair

Speaker: Dr. Johanna Brandt

RESOLUTIONS AND DISCUSSION

We hereby invite the medical authorities to send their representatives to the Meeting and to investigate our claim that we have successfully combated Cancer during the past thirty years with what is now known throughout the world as the Harmony System of Natural Healing.

A BEQUEST TO THE NATION

For the purpose of demonstrating the efficacy of this healing system, Mr. and Mrs. Fellonl, of Paarl, have endowed the nation with a beautiful farm at the foot of the Klein Drakenstein, on the main railway line in the heart of grape-growing, fruit farming and other agricultural centres.

★ Come to the City Hall on April 21st and learn about this Movement. It concerns you and the welfare of your children

ADMISSION · 1/-

Dr. Johanna Brandt's famous book on the Grape Cure for Cancer and Other Diseases, now in its fourteenth edition in the United States of America, will be for sale in the City Hall in English and Afrikaans on the 21st April.

Apply for further particulars to the Secretary,
P.O. BOX 1417, CAPE TOWN

Johanna Brandt - Notice.

The documentation of grape cures was first seen in a publication by V.N. Dmitriev called "Treatment With Grapes in Yalta on the Southern Crimean Shore" (1878). In the USSR, the principles of the grape cure were developed in the 1920s by a group of physicians of the Semashko Institute (Yalta), headed by A.V. D'iakov. Ampelotherapy continues to be offered in health clinics and spas, particularly in Europe, together with vinotherapy, a cosmetic treatment that involves rubbing grapes into the skin. Johanna Brandt, a South African doctor, popularized the grape diet as a treatment for cancer from 1925. She published about twenty pamphlets on the subject of natural remedies for health problems with her best-known publication being The Grape Cure, which is said to have been written after Brandt had cured herself of stomach cancer by following the diet. The book was republished in 1989 as How to Conquer Cancer, Naturally, including an endorsement of Brandt's work by Benedict Lust, who is commonly referred to as "the father of naturopathy". The book may have been inspired by Arnold Ehret, a contemporary, who taught a Grape Cure course.

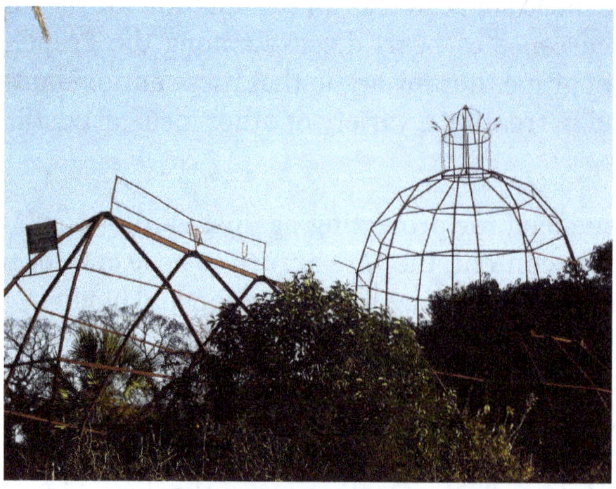

An abandoned Ampelotherapy clinic.

The leaves, stems, and grape itself, including seeds and skins, are used in herbal remedies. Most recommended diets involve large quantities of grapes, together with other foods. Treatments offered have varied from a diet that consists of eating large quantities of grapes together with other food to those that involve consuming nothing but grapes. One recommended course of ampelotherapy has to last one to two months. It is recommended to eat 2 kg (4.4 lb) of grapes with their seeds three times per week. This intake should be accompanied by a diet that limits the intake of smoked meat, milk and all dairy products and alcohol. The diet proposed by Johanna Brandt recommended fasting for two or three days, consuming only cold water, followed by a diet of only grapes and water for one to two weeks, with seven meals a day. Fresh fruits, tomatoes, and sour milk or cottage cheese are then introduced to the diet followed by raw vegetables.

Criticisms

Available scientific evidence does not support claims that a diet of grapes is alone effective for treating cancer or any other disease. Some laboratory evidence suggests that certain chemicals in grapes, their seeds and skins may help prevent heart disease and cancer, and are effective in treating diabetes but more research is needed on humans to understand the possible long-term benefits.

BENEFITS OF NATUROPATHY

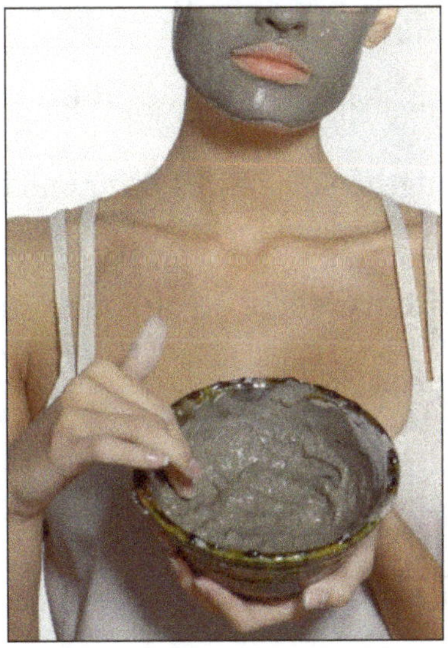

Benefits of Mud: Mud Therapy

- Mud therapy is refreshing, invigorating, and vitalizing.
- Mud therapy provides coolness as well as absorbs toxic substances from the body.
- When mud pack applied over the body for 20-30 minutes, gives reliefs from indigestion, effective in decreasing intestinal heat and stimulates peristalsis.
- Mud being a black colour absorbs all the colours of the Sun and conveys to the body.

- A thick mud pack applied to head in congestive headache relieves the pain immediately. Application of the pack over the eyes is effective for conjunctivitis, hemorrhages in the eyeball, itching, short sight and long sight.
- When soaked mud is applied on the face and allowed to dry for 30 minutes, helps to improve skin complexion, removing pimples, eliminate dark circles around eyes and open skin pores.
- Mud bath helps to improve the skin condition by increasing the circulation and energizing the skin tissues.
- For wounds and skin diseases, application of mud is the natural and true bandage.
- Mud is used successfully for diseases like constipation, headache, high blood pressure, skin diseases etc.
- The mud should be taken from 3 to 4 ft. depth from the surface of the ground to avoid contamination of chemicals, stones, debris, etc.

Benefits of Fasting for Kidney

- Fasting excretes huge amounts of accumulated wastes and poison from the body.
- The building of new cells speeded up during fasting whereas diseased, damaged, aged and dead are destroyed and eliminated.
- The eliminative power of lungs, liver, kidney and skin is greatly enhanced after fasting.
- Sugar in natural juices strengthens the heart, liver and kidney.
- Fasting gives rest to digestive, assimilative and protective organs and systems of the body thereby capacity and utilization of these organs and systems greatly enhance after fasting.
- Fasting has bigger role in diseases like indigestion, constipation, gas, digestive disorders, obesity, bp, and gout.
- The best, safest, and most effective method of fasting is lime juice fasting.

Benefits of Water: Hydro therapy

- Having bath with clean and cold water open up all the pores of the skin and make the body light and fresh.
- Cold bath activates and improves the blood circulation.
- Hydrotherapy is used mainly for preserving health and curing diseases of bilious character.
- Colon hydrotherapy washes out or detoxify colon of stagnated faecal materials and bacteria.
- Hydrotherapy helps to eliminate out undigested food and other waste products.
- Proper bath improves the natural defense mechanism or immune system of the body.

How Massage is Beneficial for you?

- Massage activates blood circulation and strengthens the body organs.
- Massage is useful high or low blood pressure, joint disorders, paralysis, depression, weakness, indigestion and obesity.
- Localized or generalized painful conditions are also getting relieved from masso therapy.
- Massage with mustard oil, sesame oil, coconut oil, olive oil, aroma oils etc. have therapeutic value. Powders of neem leaves and Rose petals are of medicinal value and used as lubricants for massage.
- Massage movements are performed through Touch, stroking, friction, kneading, vibration, percussion and joint movements.

Chromo Therapy

- Water and oil when exposed to sun for specified hours in coloured bottles or glasses, used in treating different disorders.
- Chromo therapy also helps in the recovery from different disorders.

Air Therapy

- Taking fresh air bath outside for 20 minutes is utmost important for good health.
- Air bath has soothing and tonic effect upon the millions of nerve endings of the body.
- Air bath is effective for nervousness, neurasthenia, rheumatism, skin and mental disorders.

Health Benefits of Magnet Therapy

- Magnet therapy activates the iron content in the blood and increases the RBCs and WBCs count.
- Acts like as anticoagulant and keeps the patient free blood clotting.
- Reduces the calcium and cholesterol deposits in blood.
- It helps to promote hormones secretion the body.
- It is also beneficial for the normalization of nervous system.
- For magnet therapy, therapeutic magnets, magnetic belts, magnetic necklaces, glasses and bracelets are also used for treatment.

Naturopathy Diet as Medicine

As per the norms of diet therapy, diet is divided under three sub-headings.

- Eliminative diet which includes liquids-lemon, citric juices, coconut water, vegetable soups, butter milk, etc.

- Soothing diet which comprises fruits, salads, steamed vegetables, sprouts, vegetable chutney, etc.
- Constructive diet consists of wholesome flour, unpolished rice, little pulses, sprouts, curd etc.
- Food is medicine.
- Your diet should consist of 20% acidic and 80% alkaline food for maintaining health.

NATUROPATHIC TREATMENT

Naturopathic Treatment of Obesity

Because of the complex nature of obesity, a holistic approach is often identified as best practice. Whole systems of complementary medicine (WSCAM), "complete systems of theory and practice that have evolved independently from or parallel to allopathic (conventional) medicine", can offer this type of an approach. WSCAM, including Traditional Chinese Medicine, Ayurveda, Naturopathy and classical homeopathy, are traditional historical systems of medicine that are practiced by individual cultures. These WSCAM share a perspective that imbalances in the patient's overall constitution are at the root of disease and dysfunction, including obesity. Therefore, treatment focused on the person's overall well-being would ultimately address obesity. A particular approach that is frequently used to treat obesity is Naturopathic Medicine.

Naturopathy considers obesity to be less about diet and more about correcting underlying imbalance through lifestyle change that requires a plan of care that supports long-term sustainable health optimization. Six foundational principles inform this plan and can be used to treat obesity.

Let Nature Heal

Our bodies have an innate instinct and capacity toward self-healing. By identifying and removing barriers to self-healing, such as poor diet or low self-esteem, NDs nurture this process. Patients are empowered by realizing that they are the source of healing and that external intervention is only there for support.

Identify and Treat Causes

Symptoms return unless the root illness is addressed. Rather than suppressing symptoms, NDs identify and treat their root cause. Causes of obesity are complex and multi-factorial, including factors such as lack of awareness, emotional triggers, hormone imbalance, stress, neurotransmitter imbalance, and toxicity. Therefore, treatment plans must be personalized and guidance individualized. In naturopathic medicine, health is the goal and healthy weight is an effect of being healthy. Treatment focuses on attaining overall health (e.g., regaining insulin sensitivity and reversing insulin resistance; optimal digestion; psychological well-being; decreasing stress) not on "weight loss".

First, do no Harm

Naturopathic physicians use low-risk procedures and healing compounds, such as dietary supplements, herbal extracts and homeopathy, with few or no side effects. For example, serotonin and the catecholamines (dopamine and norepinephrine) are important in the regulation of appetite and satiety. Rather than using medications such as SSRIs and phentermine, an ND might supplement a patient with amino acid precursors (5HTP for serotonin, L-tyrosine and Mucuna pruriens for dopamine and norepinephrine synthesis), thus allowing the body to make the amount of neurotransmitter it needs.

Educate Patients

A primary intervention is patient education. Teaching patients how to eat, exercise and relax/nurture themselves physically and emotionally is crucial to treatment. A naturopathic doctor might teach a patient about the "glycemic index" or "glycemic load" of foods to guide dietary choices. Alternatively, the ND may recommend the use of yoga for relaxation.

Treat the whole Person

Each individual has a unique physical, mental, emotional, genetic, environmental, social, sexual and spiritual makeup. The ND believes that all these factors contribute to health. In other words, obesity treatment is not likely to succeed unless at least psychosocial, endocrine/metabolic, and neurochemical aspects of the person are all addressed.

Prevent Illness

The primary focus of naturopathic practice is to promote health and well being, not simply to treat disease. Obesity is one of the most serious public health problems of the 21st century even though it is one of the leading causes of preventable death. NDs evaluate risk factors, heredity and vulnerability to disease. Their practice facilitates and supports lifelong lifestyle change. By addressing greater wellness, it is possible that patients will be less likely to need treatment for future illness.

Naturopathic practice is oriented to facilitate patient self-healing and use the clinical encounter as an opportunity to inspire and guide patients to develop a healthier lifestyle. Treatment of obesity is a frequent focus of ND practice. While single therapeutic agents that are used by NDs have undergone testing in research trials, to date there has been no whole-system study that supports the effectiveness of naturopathic medicine for obesity. Yet, the naturopathic philosophy of the healing, including the focus on treating the whole person and preventative care suggest that it is ideally suited for the treatment and prevention of obesity.

Naturopathic Treatment for Asthma

Asthma is a disabling disease which seriously affects the quality of life, as it weakens the capacity of the lungs to fill in oxygen. The naturopathy treatment for asthma focuses on treating the underlying causes of asthma. It is based on some key tenets like identification of the allergens, the trigger points and their prevention. Also simultaneously improving the immune system with yoga and pranayama.

Symptoms of Asthma

- Difficulty in breathing due to tensed bronchus capillaries causing a whistling sound from the ribs.

- Red and watery eyes, irritation in the feet soles and constant tiredness.
- Trouble sleeping due to frequent breathlessness, coughing at night and chest tightness.

Main Causes of Asthma

- One of the major causes of 70% of Asthma patients is allergy. Therefore, the key treatment is to identify and avoid air borne allergies like pollen and dust. And certain food like dairy, egg and gluten.
- Chronic cold is a breeding ground for Asthma. If cold is checked initially then Asthma can be prevented.
- Smoking is another main cause for Asthma. It blocks the airways to the lungs and does not let mucus to be cleaned, which damages the lungs.
- Asthma can also be hereditary. If one has a family history of Asthma then it is a high probability to inherit the disease.
- Hypertension or stress is also a major cause of Asthma. It obstructs the normal functioning of the lungs and weakens the immune system. A person suffering from hypertension sometimes experiences extreme breathlessness and the lungs fail to work properly leading to a heart attack.

Naturopathy Treatment for Asthma

In naturopathy treatments patients are given hot fomentation on the chest, back and abdomen with the help of hot water bag. They are also given mild massage on chest and back with warm mustard oil boiled with garlic cloves. Enema of lukewarm water is also recommended. Daily hot foot bath for 15 minutes. Steam bath, Sauna bath, Sun bath also help relax the body.

Placing a hot, wrung out towel over the chest can relax the breathing muscles and restore normal breathing. Steam inhalation with a few drops of eucalyptus oil in water is also very useful in case of acute asthma attack.

Lifestyle strategies-such as singing to increase diaphragmatic breathing, swimming to increase lung capacity and postural exercises that strengthen the back and open the chest are very effective.

Allergy Testing

Identifying trigger food that leads to allergies helps reduce asthma attacks.

Mucus forming foods like milk and dairy products, peanuts, citrus, banana and red meat must be avoided.

There are some environmental and lifestyle pattern that triggers asthma like pollen, animal fur, cockroach droppings, cigarette smoke, household cleaners, petrol fumes, mould and dust mites.

The most important area to focus on is the bedroom, especially crucial for kids. If possible get rid of rugs and carpets or thorough cleaning of carpets and curtains and beddings and mattress.

Diet Advised for Asthma

Diet is an integral part of naturopathy treatment, it recommends dietary changes to avoid food allergy and lessen the risk of asthma attack.

Some therapeutic food:

- Food low on fat and sugar.
- Vegetarian diet high in alkaline content such as fruits and vegetables with natural anti inflammatory nutrients such as omega-3.
- High complex carbohydrates, such as whole grains and starchy vegetables.
- Food that add moisture to the lungs such as garlic, onion, almonds, walnuts, green leafy vegetables.
- Vegetables like bottle gourd, carrot , cabbage, bitter gourd garlic, fenugreek, drumstick, carrot, lime, spinach, celery and papaya.

Yoga and Pranayam

Yoga and Pranayama are an integral part of naturopathy treatment for asthma by inducing regulation of breathing for optimum health.

- Strengthen respiratory muscles.
- Eliminate inefficient use of accessory muscles of respiration (such as abdominal or neck muscles).
- Replace forceful breathing, which compresses airways, with relaxed breathing.
- Can reduce hyperventilation by breathing exercise.
- Reduces breathlessness by increasing the functioning of the diaphragm.
- Enhances clearing of airways and gives the confidence to withstand breathlessness.

References

- Naturopathy, about-the-systems: gov.in, Retrieved 25 February, 2019
- Champeau, rachel. "antioxidant found in grapes uncorks new targets for acne treatment". Ucla newsroom. Retrieved 26 december 2014
- Salient-features-naturopathy, naturopathy, about-the-systems: gov.in, Retrieved 16 January, 2019
- Brandt, johanna (2012). The grape cure (special pocket-size ed.). Yonkers, n.y.: ehret literature publishing. Isbn 978-1570672798
- Top-and-best-medicinal-health-benefits-of-naturopathy-natural-and-herbal-treatments, health: gyanunlimited.com, Retrieved 29 March, 2019
- Naturopathy-treatment-asthma, naturopathy-treatment: natural-cure.org, Retrieved 30 April, 2019

Homeopathy

5 CHAPTER

Homeopathy is a medical practice that is based on the belief that the body can cure itself. It uses small amounts of natural products like plants and minerals to stimulate the healing process. Homeopathic dilutions and arsenic album are a few treatment derivatives used for healing. The topics elaborated in this chapter will help in gaining a better perspective about these aspects of homeopathy.

Homeopathy is a medical system based on the belief that the body can cure itself. Those who practice it use tiny amounts of natural substances, like plants and minerals. They believe these stimulate the healing process.

It was developed in the late 1700s in Germany. It's common in many European countries, but it's not quite as popular in the United States.

How does it Work?

A basic belief behind homeopathy is "like cures like." In other words, something that brings on symptoms in a healthy person can in a very small dose treat an illness with similar symptoms. This is meant to trigger the body's natural defenses.

For example, red onion makes your eyes water. That's why it's used in homeopathic remedies for allergies. Treatments for other ailments are made from poison ivy, white arsenic, crushed whole bees, and an herb called arnica.

Homeopathic doctors (who also are called "homeopaths") weaken these ingredients by adding water or alcohol. Then they shake the mixture as part of a process called "potentization." They believe this step transfers the healing essence. Homeopaths also believe that the lower the dose, the more powerful the medicine. In fact, many of these remedies no longer contain any molecules of the original substance. They come in a variety of forms, like sugar pellets, liquid drops, creams, gels, and tablets.

During your appointment, a homeopath will ask a number of questions about your mental, emotional, and physical health. He'll prescribe the remedy that best matches all of your symptoms. Then he'll tailor the treatment for you.

You can also buy over-the-counter homeopathic remedies at drugstores and health food stores. The dosage and quality of these products depend on the manufacturer.

What Conditions does Homeopathy Treat?

It's used for a wide variety of health issues, including some chronic illnesses:

- Allergies,

- Migraines,
- Depression,
- Chronic fatigue syndrome,
- Rheumatoid arthritis,
- Irritable bowel syndrome,
- Premenstrual syndrome.

It can also be used for minor issues like bruises, scrapes, toothaches, headaches, nausea, coughs, and colds.

Don't use homeopathic medicine for life-threatening illnesses, like asthma, cancer, and heart disease, or in emergencies. You should also avoid using it in place of vaccines. Some homeopathic products called "nosodes" are marketed as an alternative for vaccines, but there's no research to prove they're effective.

Homeopathy

Some studies show that homeopathic remedies are helpful, while others don't. Critics chalk up the benefits to the placebo effect. That's when symptoms improve because you believe the treatment is working not because it really is. This can trigger the brain to release chemicals that briefly relieve the pain or other symptoms.

Doctors are divided because some of the theories behind homeopathy don't line up with the principles of chemistry and physics. Scientists argue that a medicine with no active ingredient shouldn't have an effect on the body.

Importance of Homeopathy

Homeopathy is a complete medical science which compared to other systems has a clear-cut advantage as one can certainly cure psychological, pathological and physiological disorders.

In today's conventional practice, the physician spends very little time with the patient. He may listen to what is wrong with you and just give some medication for that particular suffering only. But a Homeopath will inquire into the cause behind the trouble and go up to the root of the disease. For example: Your recurring headaches may be due to some other disorder in your body such as constipation or acidity or it may be due to stress. A homeopath will aim to remove the reason behind the headaches such as constipation, etc. or inquire patiently why are you stressed and show you the way out. Homeopathy has some fine drugs to remove the effects of stress and revitalize you so that you can win over the mental stress. Once the stress is overcome, your headaches will certainly disappear forever.

Usually you may notice that Homeopaths take a detailed history of the patient. This is to dig deep and find out each small cause of all your troubles whether small or big. Often one troubling sickness may be connected to a smaller sickness not recognized by you. If that is left untouched this may also flare up. So, the Homeopath studies the entire scenario encompassing each disorder and treats you for all the trouble at a time.

Also most advantageous is that all the homeopathic drugs are derived from nature and natural substances and if used under proper supervision it will not have any side effects whatsoever.

Homeopathy cures by stimulating and restoring body's vital energy to heal itself and when this happens you will be rid of each of your troubles small or big; old or new; it protects you from future troubles too.

Homeopathy is a holistic science, which cures and heals, rather than just alleviating the symptoms of the disease, and takes into consideration the minutest details of the suffering person. In order to do this, a homeopathic physician needs to spend a substantial amount of time with the patient and understand several aspects about him and his life.

During the process of homeopathic case taking, he not only enquires about the physical ailments in detail but also questions about his general state of health, illnesses in the past and family, his life situation, anxieties and stress, fears, dreams etc. This helps the physician to perceive the diseased person in totality, thereby enabling him to find the right homeopathic similimum (exact remedy) for the patient. It also helps the patient to trust in his physician and develop a good relationship with him.

Homeopathy is natural. It is based on the law of nature - 'Law of Similars' - like cures likes. i.e. It is a method of curing the sufferings in a diseased individual by administration of remedies that have the capacity to produce similar sufferings in a relatively healthy individual (by symptom similarity). For e.g., if the symptoms of diarrhea are similar to that of poisoning by arsenic then arsenic will be your homeopathic remedy.

The homeopathic medicines are prepared from the natural substances obtained from the plant, mineral and animal kingdom.

The patient will not get fed up of taking plenty of medicines as in homeopathy only one remedy is administered at a time. No matter how many symptoms are experienced by the patient like pain in leg, cramps in stomach, giddiness etc. different remedies are not given for each of the complaint. A single remedy is administered which will exactly match to these symptoms experienced by the patient, as homeopathy treats the individual and not each symptom.

In acute conditions after administration of the medicine it will bring back the lost harmony in a rapid gentle way without producing any complications or side effects.

The homeopathic medicines do not have side effects when they are used judicially. As the action is at the dynamic level and drug substance is minimum.

Homeopathy is very safe, even for pregnant women and babies.

Homeopathic medicines can be taken along with other medications without any side effects of homeopathic medicines.

Homeopathy works in harmony with the immune system and brings back the lost balance when it is in a diseased state. When the right homeopathic medicine is administered it stimulates the body and produces an action, which is known as the primary action and then the body will take care of the disease, which is known as the secondary action.

The effect of homeopathic medicine is best seen in children. When children are put on homeopathy it allows the child to blossom like a flower and even the hereditary tendencies which run in family can be minimized. The homeopathic medicines can be administered in a very simple way and because of its sweet taste kids take the medicines without any fuss.

It does not lead to something known as drug dependency.

It improves the overall immunity of the person so he does not fall sick frequently.

In chronic diseases after the remedy is administered, it will act at a very deep level and will help the individual to fight the disease. We can get good results if the case is properly managed and if the patient commences homeopathic treatment at the onset of the sickness as it gives the original unmodified picture of his illness.

Homeopathy stimulates our immune system to fight the disease and thus does not suppress the disease. For e.g. when you take cough syrups it suppresses the cough reflex and this cough reflex is the body's attempt to clear the lungs.

Homeopathy has holistic individualistic approach; it treats all the symptoms as one, it removes the cause of the disease and thus the symptoms treated by homeopathy never recurs.

This medication can be started immediately even before the investigations are done or the diagnosis is established, thus restricting the progress of the disease and thereby decreases the structural and pathological damage occurring in the body.

Homeopathy works as a preventive and helps to maintain the healthy state of the individual not affected by the environment. In homeopathy there are medicines, which can be given as a prophylactic medicine that will help the individual to prevent the disease when other family member is suffering from a contagious disease. For e.g. if one child is suffering from chicken pox, in order to prevent the other child from getting the infection if he is given the indicated remedy he will not suffer from that disease or even if he suffers, it will be in a very mild form.

Homeopathic medicine can be very useful during epidemics. The remedy that is selected on the symptoms that are characteristic during the epidemic is known as the Genus Epidemicus. This genus epidemicus when given to the people where there is an outbreak will help the people in not contracting the epidemic disease. For e.g. Cholera, Influenza, bird flue, etc.

Homeopathy can be used for a wide range of diseases with success, if practiced in the judicial way. Let us make a healthy harmonious living possible through Homeopathy.

COMMON HOMEOPATHIC MEDICINES

Allium cepa (onion): Because it is known to cause tearing of the eyes and dripping of the nose, it is a frequent remedy for the common cold and hay fever, especially when there is a thin, watery, and burning nasal discharge that irritates the nostrils. Typically, the person's symptoms are worse in a warm room and are relieved in a cool room or in the open air.

Arnica (mountain daisy): This is a remedy in sports medicine and first aid. It is used for shock and trauma from injury. It also helps to reduce pain from injury and to speed the healing process.

Whether you're into competitive sports or exercise regularly or if you simply don't like to feel the pain of an injury, Arnica is the place to start.

Arnica (topical): The above use of Arnica is for internal consumption, usually in pill or pellet form. Another way to use Arnica is in a topical external application in a gels, ointment, or spray form. This application of Arnica is great for healing sprains and strains as well as black and blue bruising (without broken skin).

Chamomilla (chamomille): Many parents owe their sleep to homeopathy, not because it helps them directly, but because it is so good for their infant. Chamomilla is the remedy for the irritable infant, especially from teething or colic. The infant cries incessantly, and nothing seems to provide any relief, except carrying them, and even then, the crying begins recurs as soon as the parent puts the child down.

Hypericum (St. John's wort): This remedy is the first medicine to consider for injuries to the nerves or to parts of the body rich with them, including the fingers, toes, and back. Any injury with shooting pains should be given this remedy.

Ignatia (St. Ignatius bean): One day this remedy will be used by the majority of psychiatrists. It is one of the leading homeopathic medicines for acute grief, anxiety, and depression, especially after a death or separation from a loved one. The person sighs frequently, has a lump in the throat, and may tremble.

Magnesia phosphorica (phosphate of magnesia): This is the most effective remedy for cramps, including menstrual cramps. It is particularly indicated when a woman's cramps cause her to bend over and when they experience some relief from warm applications.

Nux vomica (poison nut): This is the premier medicine for ailments exacerbated by conventional or recreational drugs. It is also a common remedy for treating symptoms of overeating or from drinking too much alcohol. Considering how many people have these vices, this is an all too frequent medicine today.

Pulsatilla (windflower): Perhaps the most common remedy given to both children and women, this medicine is not indicated for a specific disease but for a specific pattern of physical symptoms and psychological characteristics. Physically, these people are warm-blooded: they wear less clothes than others, prefer open air, and don't feel as well in the heat. Psychologically, they are a gentle, mind, and yielding person, with a quickly changing emotional state and a strong tendency to want to please others.

Rhus tox (poison ivy): This medicine is the most common remedy for sprains and strains. It is especially indicated when a person experiences a "rusty gate" syndrome, that is, pain on initial motion which is reduced the more the person continues to move. It is also often given to people with the flu or arthritis who experience this similar rusty gate syndrome.

HOMEOPATHIC MATERIA MEDICA

A homeopathic materia medica is a reference guide to homeopathic medicines that describes individual active ingredients and the symptoms that they may address. A materia medica lists homeopathic ingredients in alphabetical order and provides a summary of "provings," or research, for each ingredient. A typical listing will describe the general characteristics of the substance, followed by a detailed list of symptoms associated with that substance.

In any field of medicine, the term refers to the collected body of knowledge about drugs or medications.

Samuel Hahnemann, the founder of homeopathy, was inspired while he was translating a botanical materia medica by a Scottish physician from English into German. He was intrigued by the use of Peruvian cinchona bark, which causes fever if ingested, to make quinine, a medicine used to treat fever. Hahnemann went on to establish one of the essential principles of homeopathic medicine: "Like cures like." Known as the Law of Similars, this holds that an ingredient that causes certain symptoms in a healthy person may cure similar symptoms in a sick person, when delivered in specially prepared micro-doses.

Hahnemann assembled the first homeopathic materia medica, based on research conducted in the late 18th and early 19th centuries. Since then, numerous homeopathic practitioners have written materia medica. Today, many of these documents can be accessed online. As a general term, "the homeopathic materia medica" may refer to the entire body of research and knowledge about homeopathic medications.

Homeopathic Provings

Homeopathic materia medica describe research results known as "provings." The foundational research for homeopathy was conducted when undiluted (often toxic) ingredients were tested on healthy participants called "provers." These test subjects were often homeopathic practitioners themselves, as well as their friends and family. Researchers' observations about the ill effects of these undiluted substances are known as "provings."

The symptoms listed in a typical materia medica entry actually describe the symptoms that are produced by an undiluted ingredient. Following the principle of "Like cures like," these ingredients may be expected to remedy similar symptoms, when administered in a homeopathically prepared microdose.

How to use Homeopathic Materia Medica

Homeopathic practitioners use findings from the materia medica to identify the correct medication for a given affliction. Often, practitioners will cross-reference their findings with another type of document called a repertory. Whereas a materia medica starts with the medicine and lists associated symptoms, a repertory starts with the symptom and lists applicable medicines.

It is not recommended for people without substantial training in homeopathy to use materia medica and repertories to select homeopathic treatments. Application of these reference documents is an advanced skill, which requires understanding of, among other things, the terminology used in these classical texts, names and abbreviations for ingredients, and subtle variations in symptoms.

HOMEOPATHIC DILUTIONS

In homeopathy, homeopathic dilution (known by practitioners as "dynamisation" or "potentisation") is a process in which a substance is diluted with alcohol or distilled water and then vigorously shaken in a process called "succussion". Insoluble solids, such as quartz and oyster shell, are diluted by grinding them with lactose (trituration). The founder of homeopathy, Samuel Hahnemann believed that the process of succussion activated the "vital energy" of the diluted substance, and that successive dilutions increased the "potency" of the preparation, although other strands of homeopathy disagree.

The concept is pseudoscience because, at commonly used dilutions, no molecules of the original material are likely to remain.

Potency Scales

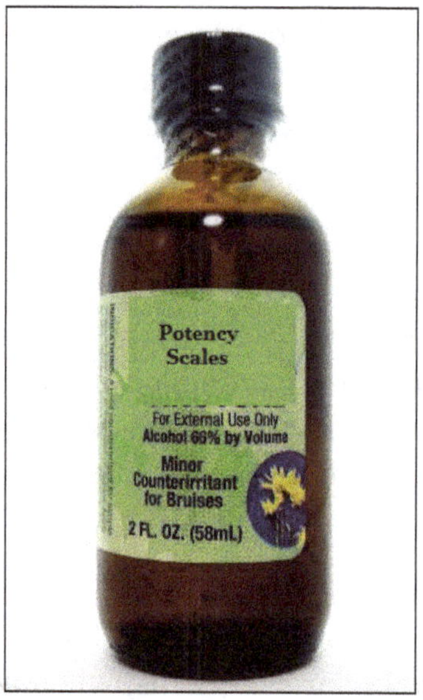

This bottle contains Arnica montana D6, i.e. the nominal dilution is one part in a million.

Several potency scales are in use in homeopathy. Hahnemann created the centesimal or "C scale", diluting a substance by a factor of 100 at each stage. The centesimal scale was favored by Hahnemann for most of his life. A 2C dilution requires a substance to be diluted to one part in one hundred, and then some of that diluted solution diluted by a further factor of one hundred. This works out to one part of the original substance in 10,000 parts of the solution. A 6C dilution repeats this process six times, ending up with the original material diluted by a factor of $100^{-6}=10^{-12}$. Higher dilutions follow the same pattern. In homeopathy, a solution that is more dilute is described as having a higher potency, and more dilute substances are considered by homeopaths to be stronger and deeper-acting. The end product is often so diluted that it is indistinguishable from the dilutant (typically ethanol or pure water for liquids, milk sugar for insoluble solids).

Hahnemann advocated 30C dilutions for most purposes (that is, dilution by a factor of 10^{60}). In Hahnemann's time it was reasonable to assume that preparations could be diluted indefinitely, as the concept of the atom or molecule as the smallest possible unit of a chemical substance was just beginning to be recognized. We now know that the greatest dilution that is reasonably likely to contain one molecule of the original substance is 12C, if starting from 1 mole of original substance.

Some homeopaths developed a decimal scale (D or X), diluting the substance to ten times its original volume each stage. The D or X scale dilution is therefore half that of the same value of the C scale; for example, "12X" is the same level of dilution as "6C". Hahnemann never used this scale but it was very popular throughout the 19th century and still is in Europe. This potency scale appears to have been introduced in the 1830s by the American homeopath Constantine Hering. In the last ten years of his life, Hahnemann also developed a quintamillesimal (Q) or LM scale diluting the drug 1 part in 50,000 parts of diluent. A given dilution on the Q scale is roughly 2.35 times its designation on the C scale. For example, a preparation described as "20Q" has about the same concentration as one described with "47C"g.

Potencies of 1000C and above are usually labelled with Roman numeral M and with the centesimal 'C' indicator implied (since all such high potencies are centesimal dilutions): 1M = 1000C; 10M = 10,000C; CM = 100,000C; LM (which would indicate 50,000C) is typically not used because of confusion with the LM potency scale.

The following table is a synopsis comparing the X and C dilution scales and equating them by equivalent dilution. However, the homeopathic understanding of its principles is not explained by dilution but by "potentisation", hence one can not assume that the different potencies can be equated on the basis of equivalence of dilution factors.

X Scale	C Scale	Ratio	Note
1X	–	1:10	described as low potency
2X	1C	1:100	called higher potency than 1X by homeopaths
6X	3C	10^{-6}	
8X	4C	10^{-8}	
12X	6C	10^{-12}	
24X	12C	10^{-24}	Has a 60% probability of containing one molecule of original material if one mole of the original substance was used.
26X	13C	10^{-26}	If pure water were used as the diluent, no molecules of the original solution remain in the water.
60X	30C	10^{-60}	Dilution advocated by Hahnemann for most purposes: on average, this would require giving two billion doses per second to six billion people for 4 billion years to deliver a single molecule of the original material to any patient.
400X	200C	10^{-400}	Dilution of popular homeopathic flu preparation Oscillococcinum
Note: the "X scale" is also called "D scale". 1X = 1D, 2X = 2D, etc.			

Dilutions

Serial dilution of a solution results, after each dilution step, in fewer molecules of the original substance per litre of solution. Eventually, a solution will be diluted beyond any likelihood of finding a single molecule of the original substance in a litre of the total dilution product.

The Molar Limit

If one begins with a solution of 1 mol/L of a substance, the dilution required to reduce the number of molecules to less than one per litre is 1 part in 1×10^{24} (24X or 12C) since:

$$6.02 \times 10^{23} / 1 \times 10^{24} = 0.6 \text{ molecules per litre}$$

Homeopathic dilutions beyond this limit (equivalent to approximately 12C) are unlikely to contain a single molecule of the original substance and lower dilutions contain no detectable amount. ISO 3696 (Water for analytical laboratory use) specifies a purity of ten parts per billion, or 10×10^{-9} – this water cannot be kept in glass or plastic containers as they leach impurities into the water, and glassware must be washed with hydrofluoric acid before use. Ten parts per billion is equivalent to a homeopathic dilution of 4C.

Analogies

Critics and advocates of homeopathy alike commonly attempt to illustrate the dilutions involved in homeopathy with analogies. The high dilutions characteristically used are often considered to be the most controversial and implausible aspect of homeopathy.

A popular homeopathic treatment for the flu is a 200C dilution of duck liver, marketed under the name Oscillococcinum. As there are only about 10^{80} atoms in the entire observable universe, a dilution of one molecule in the observable universe would be about 40C. Oscillococcinum would thus require 10^{320} times more atoms to simply have one molecule in the final substance.

Another illustration of dilutions used in common homeopathic preparations involves comparing a homeopathic dilution to dissolving the therapeutic substance in a swimming pool. There are on the order of 10^{32} molecules of water in an Olympic-size swimming pool and if such a pool were filled entirely with a 15C homeopathic preparation, to have a 63% chance of consuming at least one molecule of the original substance, one would need to swallow 1% of the volume of such a pool, or roughly 25 metric tons of water.

Proposed Explanations

Homeopaths maintain that this water retains some "essential property" of the original material, because the preparation has been shaken after each dilution. Hahnemann believed that the dynamisation or shaking of the solution caused a "spirit-like" healing force to be released from within the substance. Even though the homeopathic preparations are often extremely diluted, homeopaths maintain that a healing force is retained by these homeopathic preparations. Modern advocates of homeopathy have proposed a concept of "water memory", according to which water "remembers" the substances mixed in it, and transmits the effect of those substances when consumed. This concept is inconsistent with the current understanding of matter, and water memory has never been demonstrated to have any detectable effect, biological or otherwise. The claim often given to support "water memory" is that science does not fully understand water. In fact a great deal is known about the structure and properties of liquid water, from both theoretical and experimental studies, because of its importance in biochemistry, its relative molecular simplicity and the quantum mechanical nature of hydrogen bonding which make it a popular substance to study in theoretical chemistry. The actual memory of water can be measured experimentally and is found to be around 50 femtoseconds, which is 0.00000000000005 seconds. Generally considered to be pseudoscience by the scientific community, one disputed study into the so-called memory of water, conducted by Jacques Benveniste, claims to have demonstrated that water can be energetically imprinted upon. Another such study, published in 2003 by Swiss chemist Louis Rey, claims to have found that homeopathically diluted solutions of sodium chloride and lithium chloride have a very different hydrogen bond structure from normal water, as measured by thermoluminescence.

Dilution Debate

Not all homeopaths advocate extremely high dilutions. Many of the early homeopaths were originally doctors and generally used lower dilutions such as "3X" or "6X", rarely going beyond "12X"; these dilution ("trituration") levels were still popular in the late 20th century with advocates of Wilhelm Heinrich Schüßler's 12 biochemic tissue salts, for example. The split between lower and higher dilutions followed ideological lines. Those favoring low dilutions stressed pathology and a strong link to conventional medicine, while those favoring high dilutions emphasised vital force, miasms and a spiritual interpretation of disease. Some products with both low and high dilutions continue to be sold, but like their counterparts, they have not been conclusively demonstrated to have any effect when tested against placebo.

ELECTROHOMEOPATHY

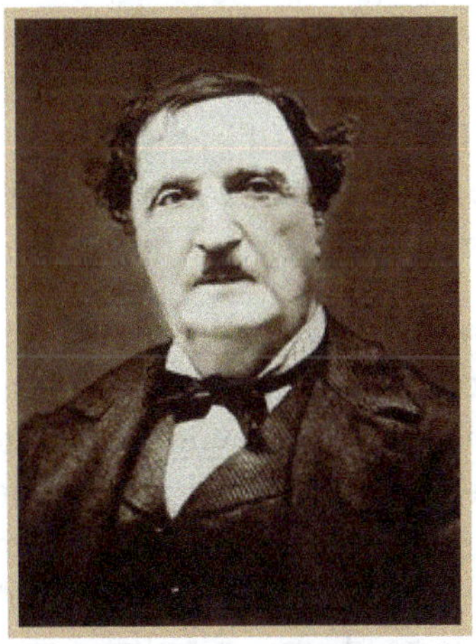

Count Cesare Mattei.

Electrohomoeopathy (or Mattei cancer cure) is a derivative of homeopathy invented in the 19th century by Count Cesare Mattei. The name is derived from a combination of electro (referring to an electric bio-energy content supposedly extracted from plants and of therapeutic value, rather than electricity in its conventional sense) and homeopathy (referring to an alternative medicinal philosophy developed by Samuel Hahnemann in the 18th century). Electrohomeopathy has been defined as the combination of electrical devices and homeopathy.

Lucrative for its inventor and popular in the late nineteenth century, electrohomoeopathy has been described as "utter idiocy". Like all homeopathy, it is regarded by the medical and scientific communities as pseudoscience and its practice as quackery.

Electrohomeopathy was devised by Cesare Mattei in the latter part of the 19th century. Mattei, a nobleman living in a castle in the vicinity of Bologna, studied natural science, anatomy, physiology, pathology, chemistry and botany. He ultimately focused on the supposed therapeutic power of "electricity" in botanical extracts. Mattei made bold, unsupported claims for the efficacy of his treatments, including the claim that his treatments offered a nonsurgical alternative to cancer. His treatment regimens were met with scepticism by mainstream medicine:

> The electrohomeopathic system is an invention of Count Mattei who prates of "red", "yellow" and "blue", "green" and "white" electricity, a theory that, in spite of its utter idiocy, has attracted a considerable following and earned a large fortune for its chief promoter.

Notwithstanding criticisms, including a challenge by the British medical establishment to the claimed success of his cancer treatments, electrohomeopathy (or Matteism, as it was sometimes known at the time) had adherents in Germany, France, the USA and the UK by the beginning of the 20th century; electrohomeopathy had been the subject of approximately 100 publications and there were three journals dedicated to it.

Remedies are derived from what are said to be the active micro nutrients or mineral salts of certain plants. One contemporary account of the process of producing electrohomeopathic remedies was as follows:

> As to the nature of his remedies we learn that they are manufactured from certain herbs, and that the directions for the preparation of the necessary dilutions are given in the ordinary jargon of homeopathy. The globules and liquids, however, are "instinct with a potent, vital, electrical force, which enables them to work wonders". This process of "fixing the electrical principle" is carried on in the secret central chamber of a Neo-Moorish castle which Count Mattei has built for himself in the Bolognese Apennines. The "red electricity" and "white electricity" supposed to be "fixed" in these "vegetable compounds" are in their very nomenclature and suggestion poor and miserable fictions.

According to Mattei's own ideas however, every disease originates in the change of blood or of the lymphatic system or both, and remedies can therefore be mainly divided into two broad categories to be used in response to the dominant affected system. Mattei wrote that having obtained plant extracts, he was "able to determine in the liquid vegetable electricity". Allied to his theories and therapies were elements of Chinese medicine, of medical humours, of apparent Brownianism, as well as modified versions of Samuel Hahnemann's homeopathic principles. Electrohomeopathy has some associations with Spagyric medicine, a holistic medical philosophy claimed to be the practical application of alchemy in medical treatment, so that the principle of modern electrohomeopathy is that disease is typically multi-organic in cause or effect and therefore requires holistic treatment that is at once both complex and natural.

Modern Usage

A symposium took place in Bologna in 2008 to mark the 200th anniversary of the birth of Cesare Mattei, with attendees from India, Pakistan, Germany, UK, and the USA. Electrohomeopathy is practiced predominantly in India and Pakistan (RAJYA SABHA Parliamentary Bulletin- The Recognition of Electro Homeopathy System of Medicine Bill, 2015 by E. M. Sudarsana Natchiappan, M. P), but there are also a number of electrohomeopathy organizations and institutions worldwide.

ARSENICUM ALBUM

Arsenic is a toxic chemical element, historically used as a poison. It is safe to use with infants through to the elderly when prepared in homeopathic potencies. Those who need Arsenicum are prone to hypochondriasis and are intolerant of untidiness and disorder. They are anxious, critical, and restless, and dislike being alone but may be irritable with company. Restlessness may be followed by exhaustion which is out of proportion to their illness. They fear illness and disease, death, and being alone. Discharges tend to be acrid and burning. Burning pains paradoxically feel better for heat (except the headache which is better for cold applications). Thirst is for sips of warm drinks but cold drinks worsen. Symptoms worsen between midnight and 2 AM.

Colds and Hayfever

- Red, puffy, burning eyes that feel better for hot compresses.
- Watery, nasal discharge that burns and reddens the nostrils and lip.
- Frequent sneezing with no relief.

Coughs

- Worsened by cold air or cold drinks.
- Rapid, difficult breathing, with wheezing (asthma).
- Coughs or wheezing worse for lying down and better for sitting upright headaches.
- Burning, throbbing pain.
- Worsened by heat and relieved by cold applications or cool air (though rest of body will be chilly and rugged up).

Skin Problems

- Eczema with burning, itching, dry skin.

Digestive Problems

- Thirst for frequent small sips of water.
- Burning stomach pains eased by drinking milk.
- Offensive, burning, scalding diarrhoea.
- A key remedy for food poisoning or gastroenteritis.

Fever

- Hot head and cold body.
- Chilly and want to be rugged up.

Sleep

- Restless and anxious – insomnia between midnight and 2 AM.
- Dreams of robbers.

For Pets

- Chilly, anxious pets.
- Itchy, dry skin eruptions in chilly, anxious animals.

Important

While above self-limiting or acute complaints are suitable for home treatment, see your healthcare provider if symptoms worsen or fail to improve. Chronic or persistent complaints, require a different treatment and dosage protocol so are best managed by a qualified homeopath for good results.

Dosage Instructions

For acute and self-limiting complaints, take one pill or five drops of the remedy every 30 minutes to 4 hours (30 minutes for intense symptoms, 4 hours for milder ones). Once an improvement is noticed, stop dosing and repeat the remedy only if symptoms return. If there is no improvement at all by three doses, choose a different remedy or seek professional guidance. Chronic symptoms or complaints require a course of professional treatment to manage the changes in potencies and remedies that will be required.

References

- What-is-homeopathy, balance: webmd.com, Retrieved 29 June, 2019
- Advantages-of-homeopathy: specialityclinic.com, Retrieved 14 July, 2019
- Grimes, D. R. (2012). "Proposed mechanisms for homeopathy are physically impossible". Focus on Alternative and Complementary Therapies. 17 (3): 149–155. doi:10.1111/j.2042-7166.2012.01162.x
- Ten-common-homeopathic-medicines: homeopathic.com
- Kayne SB (2006), Homeopathic pharmacy: theory and practice (2 ed.), Elsevier Health Sciences, p. 53, ISBN 978-0-443-10160-1
- Homeopathic-materia-medica-3, homeopathy, about-arnica: arnica.com, Retrieved 11 January, 2019
- Robert L. Park (2008). Superstition: Belief in the Age of Science. Princeton University Press. pp. 145–146. ISBN 978-0-691-13355-3
- Know-your-remedies-arsenicum-album-ars: homeopathyplus.com, Retrieved 31 March, 2019

Important Therapies in Alternative Medicine

CHAPTER 6

There are various important therapies in alternative medicines such as acupressure, auriculotherapy, acupuncture, apitherapy, hypnotherapy, detoxification, ozone therapy, balneotherapy, halotherapy, etc. This chapter has been carefully written to provide an easy understanding of these therapies of alternative medicine.

ACUPRESSURE

Acupressure is an alternative medicine technique similar in principle to acupuncture.

It is based on the concept of life energy which flows through "meridians" in the body. In treatment, physical pressure is applied to points with the aim of clearing blockages in these meridians. Pressure may be applied by hand, by elbow, or with various devices.

The points are commonly called "acupuncture points," "pressure points," "acupoints" or "acupressure points."

Traditional Chinese medical theory describes special acupoints or acupressure points, that lie along meridians, or channels, in your body. These are the same energy meridians and acupoints as those targeted with acupuncture. It is believed that through these invisible channels flows vital energy or a life force called qi (ch'i). It is also believed that these 12 major meridians connect specific organs or networks of organs, organizing a system of communication throughout your body. The meridians begin at your fingertips, connect to your brain, and then connect to an organ associated with a certain meridian.

According to this theory, when one of these meridians is blocked or out of balance, illness can occur. Acupressure and acupuncture are among the types of TCM that are thought to help restore balance.

Acupressure Techniques: Pressing and Reducing points

There are two ways that acupressure points are manipulated: pressing (reinforcing) and reducing them. Most are probably familiar with the first, but not with the second method.

- Pressing points: Usually the fingers are used to press, but fingers may be a bit too thick, so you'd have to press quite long and firmly. Ideal would be something 3 to 4 mm thick, like a (preferably used) pencil eraser that's on the other side of a pencil. Some points can be pressed using a fingernail. Pressing points for less than half a second can already have a distinguishable effect. To get a full effect however, pressure should be applied for at least half a minute, but preferably longer. One to two minutes should do.

- Reducing: To reduce a point, turn a finger over it in counter-clockwise direction, also for one to two minutes.

We spoke little about acupressure in previous and now we continue.Acupressure points, like reflexology points in the soles of the feet, are described as areas of the skin where meridians or channels terminate from connections to various parts of the body.

These meridians provide a circulation system for electrical energy throughout the body and can be thought of as a communications network. Simply, they can be used to direct the body's nervous system to release muscular tension and assist the flow of blood to injured parts.

It is thought that negative magnetic energy plays a major role in this process within the body and the use of negative magnetic stimulus externally can be most effective.

What is Magnet Therapy?

When acupoints are used with Magnets, it is called as 'Magnet therapy'.In Magnet therapy, very small magnets are placed on acupoints which help in restoring the bioenergetic balance.They are sometimes attached by placing them underneath an elastic bandage, or taping them into position using medical tape made of a comfortable fabric.

As a result of such effects, magnet therapy can function as an antibiotic, eliminating many microbes, viruses, bacteria, and fungi, including strains which may be resistant to pharmaceutical antibiotics or other drugs.

Recently, it has also been discovered that the cells of the brain themselves contain a substance called magnetite. Magnetite is a naturally occurring crystalline material with weak magnetic properties, and which receives its charge from the Earth's magnetic field. As a result of these mechanics, applying a therapeutic magnet to the head stimulates production of the hormone melatonin, thereby improving the quality of sleep, balancing the person's sleep cycle, and otherwise facilitating relaxation and altered states of consciousness.

Ways to use Acupressure

- The applications of using acupressure include relieving pain, balancing body energy, and maintaining good health.
- Acupressure's healing touch reduces muscular tension, increases circulation, and enables deep relaxation.

Benefits and uses of Acupressure

Uses

Most people try acupressure for the first time to manage symptoms of a condition, such as:

- Cancer-related fatigue,

- Headache,
- Menstrual cramps,
- Motion sickness,
- Muscle tension and pain,
- Nausea or vomiting after surgery or chemotherapy,
- Nausea and vomiting during pregnancy and morning sickness,
- Stress management.

Benefits

There's currently a lack of studies exploring the effectiveness of acupressure. Still, there's some evidence suggesting that wrist acupressure may help to relieve pain after a sports injury. researchers examined the effects of three minutes of acupressure, three minutes of sham acupressure, or no acupressure in athletes who had sustained a sports injury on the same day.

At the study's end, acupressure was found to be effective in reducing pain intensity compared to sham acupressure or no acupressure. There was no change in anxiety.

Acupressure may help to ease nausea and vomiting in those with chemotherapy-induced nausea and vomiting.

Researchers analyzed the results of three previously published trials and found that acupressure (using finger pressure or an acupressure wristband) decreased nausea, vomiting, and retching.

AURICULOTHERAPY

Auriculotherapy (also auricular therapy, ear acupuncture, and auriculoacupuncture) is a form of alternative medicine based on the idea that the ear is a micro system, which reflects the entire body, represented on the auricle, the outer portion of the ear. Conditions affecting the physical, mental or emotional health of the patient are assumed to be treatable by stimulation of the surface of the ear exclusively. Similar mappings are used in many areas of the body, including the practices of reflexology and iridology. These mappings are not based on or supported by any medical or scientific evidence, and are therefore considered to be pseudoscience.

The oldest record of auriculotherapy dates back approximately 2500 to The Yellow Emperor's Classic of Internal Medicine (ca. 100 BCE), though it has mostly been limited to bloodletting and cauterization. For instance, chapter 63 of Plain Questions of The Yellow Emperor's Classic (Huang Di Nei Jing) refers to blowing air into the ear with a tube to save an unconscious patient. Chapter 20 of Miraculous Pivot of The Yellow Emperor's Classic mentioned phlebotomy of distended vein in the ear to relieve tightness in the costal regions.

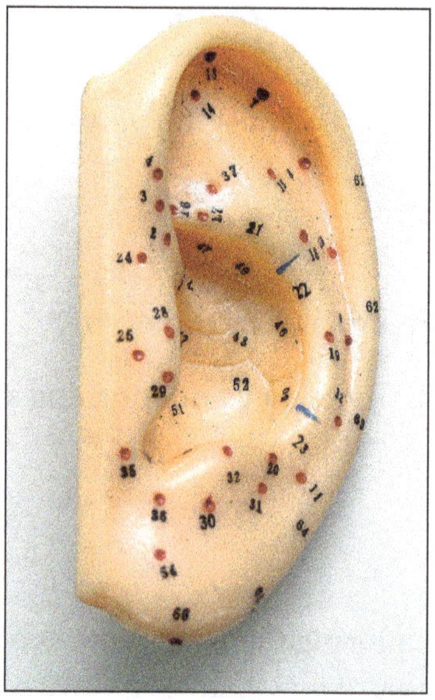

Acupuncture points in the ear.

Auriculotherapy was introduced to Europe after 1957, when French neurologist Paul Nogier proposed a more systemic and standardized approach to auriculotherapy in the "Treatise of Auriculotherapy" (1957). Auriculotherapy has since then been introduced to the international scientific community as Nogier's report has been read by Russian, Japanese, and Chinese acupuncturists, and been translated into Chinese in 1958.

The developments were made by clinical trials based upon a phrenological method of projection of a fetal Homunculus on the ear, for reference of physical complaints and points for medical treatment. Nogier soon presented his discovery to the public, where members of the Chinese Army picked up the map and took it to the barefoot doctors of China, farmers with minimal training in basic medical and in paramedical skills, and so provide medical services in rural China.

Moreover, Nogier then published what he called the "Vascular Autonomic Signal", a distinct change in the amplitude of the pulse, easily felt with the tip of the thumb at the radial artery. That mechanism would only produce a signal upon the introduction of new information to the electromagnetic field of the patient. Nogier then was working with the principle of matching resonance, and said that he could use the vascular autonomic signal to detect the active points of the auricular microsystem.

Auricular acupuncture has progressed since then, and several national programmes are being developed.

More recent development of auriculotherapy includes the emergence of a new therapy developed by Dr. Richard Niemtzow in 2001, which he coined Battlefield Acupuncture. It involves placing gold aiguille semi-permanent needles at up to five sites in the ears. He developed the Battlefield Acupuncture system in an attempt to research more efficient relief for phantom limb pain and chronic pain for veterans. The United States Department of Defense, the Veterans Center for Integrative Pain Management, and the Veterans Health Administration National Pain Management Program office recently completed a 3-year $5.4 million acupuncture education and training program, which trained over 2800 providers for Battlefield Acupuncture.

Anatomical Structures of the Auricular Surface

It is important to understand the anatomical structures of the auricle in order to locate the auricular points. The main anatomical structures include:

- Helix, the outer, prominent rim of the auricle.
    - Helix crus, a transverse ridge of helix.
- Antihelix, the elevated ridge anterior and parallel to the helix, of which the upper part branches into.
    - Superior antihelix crus: superior branch of bifurcation of the antihelix.
    - Inferior antihelix crus: inferior branch of bifurcation of the antihelix.
- Triangular fossa, the triangular depression between the two crura of the antihelix.
- Scapha, the narrow curved depression between the helix and the antihelix.
- Tragus, the small, curved flap in front of the auricle.
- Antitragus, the small tubercle opposite to the tragus.
- Concha: The hollow next to the ear canal, which is split into.
    - Cymba concha: the concha superior to the helix crus.
    - Cavum concha: the concha inferior to the helix crus.

Distribution of Auricular Points

Points located on the ear lobe are related to the head and facial region, those on the scapha are related to the upper limbs, while those on the antihelix and anihelix crura to the trunk and lower limbs, and those in the concha are related to the internal organs.

ACUPUNCTURE

Acupuncture is a form of alternative medicine and a key component of traditional Chinese medicine (TCM) in which thin needles are inserted into the body. Acupuncture is a pseudoscience because the theories and practices of TCM are not based on scientific knowledge, and it has been characterized as quackery. There is a range of acupuncture variants which originated in different philosophies, and techniques vary depending on the country in which it is performed. It is most often used to attempt pain relief, though it is also recommended by acupuncturists for a wide range of other conditions. Acupuncture is generally used only in combination with other forms of treatment.

The conclusions of numerous trials and systematic reviews of acupuncture are inconsistent, which suggests that it is not effective. An overview of Cochrane reviews found that acupuncture is not effective for a wide range of conditions. A systematic review conducted by medical scientists at the Universities of Exeter and Plymouth found little evidence of acupuncture's effectiveness in treating pain. Overall, the evidence suggests that short-term treatment with acupuncture does not produce long-term benefits. Some research results suggest that acupuncture can alleviate some forms of pain, though the majority of research suggests that acupuncture's apparent effects are not caused by the treatment itself. A systematic review concluded that the analgesic effect of acupuncture seemed to lack clinical relevance and could not be clearly distinguished from bias. One meta-analysis found that acupuncture for chronic low back pain was cost-effective as an adjunct to standard care, while a separate systematic review found insufficient evidence for the cost-effectiveness of acupuncture in the treatment of chronic low back pain.

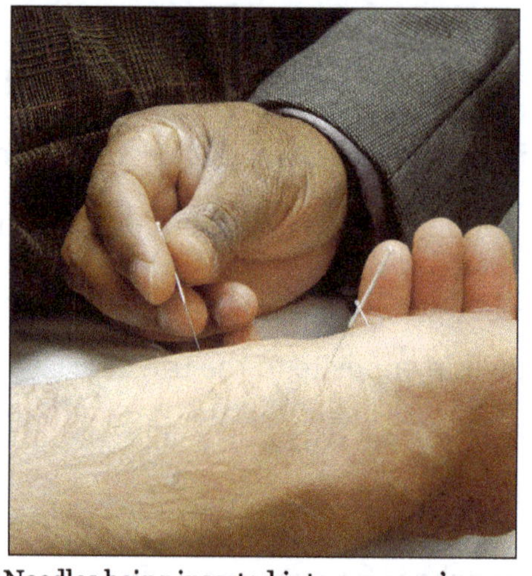

Needles being inserted into a person's arm.

Acupuncture is generally safe when done by appropriately trained practitioners using clean needle technique and single-use needles. When properly delivered, it has a low rate of mostly minor adverse effects. Accidents and infections do occur, though, and are associated with neglect on the part of the practitioner, particularly in the application of sterile techniques. A review conducted in 2013 stated that reports of infection transmission increased significantly in the preceding decade. The most frequently reported adverse events were pneumothorax and infections. Since serious adverse events continue to be reported, it is recommended that acupuncturists be trained sufficiently to reduce the risk.

Scientific investigation has not found any histological or physiological evidence for traditional Chinese concepts such as qi, meridians, and acupuncture points and many modern practitioners no longer support the existence of life force energy (qi) or meridians, which was a major part of early belief systems. Acupuncture is believed to have originated around 100 BC, around the time The Yellow Emperor's Classic of Internal Medicine (Huangdi Neijing) was published, though some experts suggest it could have been practiced earlier. Over time, conflicting claims and belief systems emerged about the effect of lunar, celestial and earthly cycles, yin and yang energies, and a body's "rhythm" on the effectiveness of treatment. Acupuncture fluctuated in popularity due to changes in the country's political leadership and the preferential use of rationalism or Western medicine. Acupuncture spread first to Korea in the 6th century AD, then to Japan through medical missionaries, and then to Europe, beginning with France. In the 20th century, as it spread to the United States and Western countries, spiritual elements of acupuncture that conflict with Western beliefs were sometimes abandoned in favor of simply tapping needles into acupuncture points.

Clinical Practice

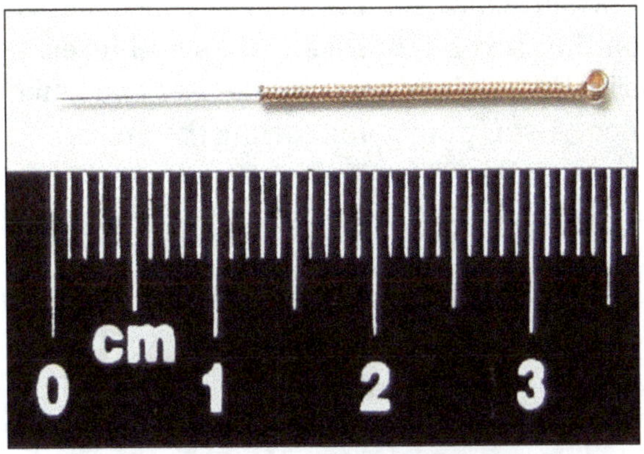

One type of acupuncture needle.

Acupuncture is a form of alternative medicine. It is used most commonly for pain relief, though it is also used to treat a wide range of conditions. Acupuncture is generally only used in combination with other forms of treatment. For example, it may be considered in the treatment for nonspecific, noninflammatory low back pain only in conjunction with conventional therapy.

Acupuncture is the insertion of thin needles into the skin. According to the Mayo Foundation for Medical Education and Research (Mayo Clinic), a typical session entails lying still while approximately five to twenty needles are inserted; for the majority of cases, the needles will be left in place for ten to twenty minutes. It can be associated with the application of heat, pressure, or laser light. Classically, acupuncture is individualized and based on philosophy and intuition, and not on scientific research. There is also a non-invasive therapy developed in early 20th century Japan using an elaborate set of "needles" for the treatment of children (*shōnishin* or *shōnihari*).

Clinical practice varies depending on the country. A comparison of the average number of patients treated per hour found significant differences between China (10) and the United States (1.2). Chinese herbs are often used. There is a diverse range of acupuncture approaches, involving different philosophies. Although various different techniques of acupuncture practice have emerged, the method used in traditional Chinese medicine (TCM) seems to be the most widely adopted in the US. Traditional acupuncture involves needle insertion, moxibustion, and cupping therapy, and may be accompanied by other procedures such as feeling the pulse and other parts of the body and examining the tongue. Traditional acupuncture involves the belief that a "life force" (*qi*) circulates within the body in lines called meridians. The main methods practiced in the UK are TCM and Western medical acupuncture. The term Western medical acupuncture is used to indicate an adaptation of TCM-based acupuncture which focuses less on TCM. The Western medical acupuncture approach involves using acupuncture after a medical diagnosis. Limited research has compared the contrasting acupuncture systems used in various countries for determining different acupuncture points and thus there is no defined standard for acupuncture points.

In traditional acupuncture, the acupuncturist decides which points to treat by observing and questioning the patient to make a diagnosis according to the tradition used. In TCM, the four diagnostic methods are: inspection, auscultation and olfaction, inquiring, and palpation. Inspection focuses on the face and particularly on the tongue, including analysis of the tongue size, shape, tension, color and coating, and the absence or presence of teeth marks around the edge. Auscultation and olfaction involve listening for particular sounds such as wheezing, and observing body odor. Inquiring involves focusing on the "seven inquiries": chills and fever; perspiration; appetite, thirst and taste; defecation and urination; pain; sleep; and menses and leukorrhea. Palpation is focusing on feeling the body for tender *"A-shi"* points and feeling the pulse.

Needles

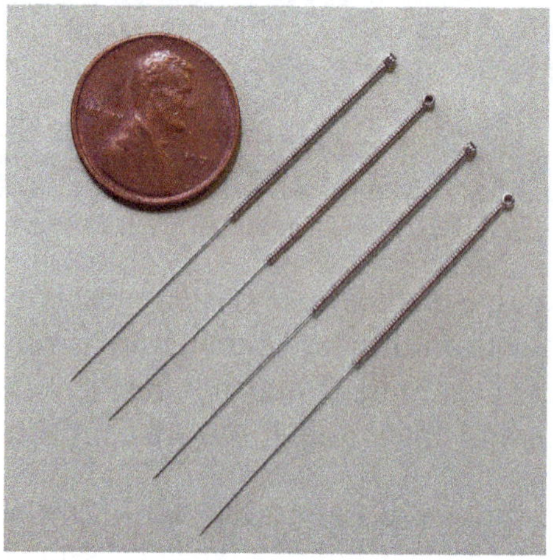

Acupuncture needles.

The most common mechanism of stimulation of acupuncture points employs penetration of the skin by thin metal needles, which are manipulated manually or the needle may be further stimulated by electrical stimulation (electroacupuncture). Acupuncture needles are typically made of stainless steel, making them flexible and preventing them from rusting or breaking. Needles are usually disposed of after each use to prevent contamination. Reusable needles when used should be sterilized between applications. Needles vary in length between 13 to 130 millimetres (0.51 to 5.12 in), with shorter needles used near the face and eyes, and longer needles in areas with thicker tissues; needle diameters vary from 0.16 mm (0.006 in) to 0.46 mm (0.018 in), with thicker needles used on more robust patients. Thinner needles may be flexible and require tubes for insertion. The tip of the needle should not be made too sharp to prevent breakage, although blunt needles cause more pain.

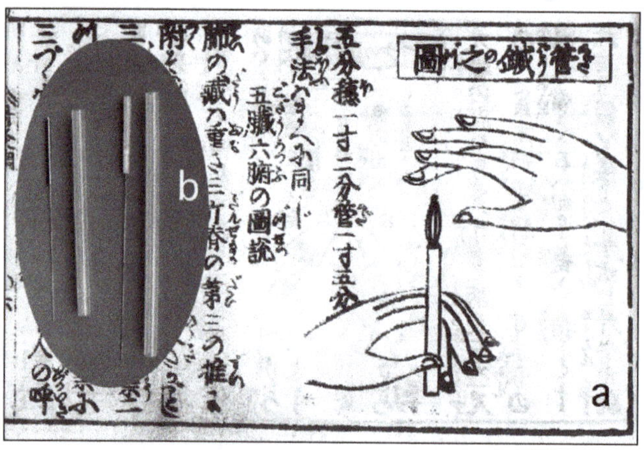

Traditional and modern Japanese guiding tube needles.

Apart from the usual filiform needle, other needle types include three-edged needles and the Nine Ancient Needles. Japanese acupuncturists use extremely thin needles that are used superficially, sometimes without penetrating the skin, and surrounded by a guide tube (a 17th-century invention adopted and the West). Korean acupuncture uses copper needles and has a greater focus on the hand.

Needling Technique

Insertion

The skin is sterilized and needles are inserted, frequently with a plastic guide tube. Needles may be manipulated in various ways, including spinning, flicking, or moving up and down relative to the skin. Since most pain is felt in the superficial layers of the skin, a quick insertion of the needle is recommended. Often the needles are stimulated by hand in order to cause a dull, localized, aching sensation that is called *de qi*, as well as "needle grasp," a tugging feeling felt by the acupuncturist and generated by a mechanical interaction between the needle and skin. Acupuncture can be painful. The skill level of the acupuncturist may influence how painful the needle insertion is, and a sufficiently skilled practitioner may be able to insert the needles without causing any pain.

De-qi Sensation

De-qi refers to a claimed sensation of numbness, distension, or electrical tingling at the needling site. If these sensations are not observed then inaccurate location of the acupoint, improper depth of needle insertion, inadequate manual manipulation, are blamed. If de-qi is not immediately observed upon needle insertion, various manual manipulation techniques are often applied to promote it (such as "plucking", "shaking" or "trembling").

Once de-qi is observed, techniques might be used which attempt to "influence" the de-qi; for example, by certain manipulation the de-qi can allegedly be conducted from the needling site towards more distant sites of the body. Other techniques aim at "tonifying" or "sedating" qi. The former techniques are used in deficiency patterns, the latter in excess patterns. De qi is more important in Chinese acupuncture, while Western and Japanese patients may not consider it a necessary part of the treatment.

Related Practices

- Acupressure, a non-invasive form of bodywork, uses physical pressure applied to acupressure points by the hand or elbow, or with various devices.
- Acupuncture is often accompanied by moxibustion, the burning of cone-shaped preparations of moxa (made from dried mugwort) on or near the skin, often but not always near or on an acupuncture point. Traditionally, acupuncture was used to treat acute conditions while moxibustion was used for chronic diseases. Moxibustion could be direct (the cone was placed directly on the skin and allowed to burn the skin, producing a blister and eventually a scar), or indirect (either a cone of moxa was placed on a slice of garlic, ginger or other vegetable, or a cylinder of moxa was held above the skin, close enough to either warm or burn it).

- Cupping therapy is an ancient Chinese form of alternative medicine in which a local suction is created on the skin; practitioners believe this mobilizes blood flow in order to promote healing.
- Tui na is a TCM method of attempting to stimulate the flow of *qi* by various bare-handed techniques that do not involve needles.
- Electroacupuncture is a form of acupuncture in which acupuncture needles are attached to a device that generates continuous electric pulses (this has been described as "essentially transdermal electrical nerve stimulation tens masquerading as acupuncture").
- Fire needle acupuncture also known as fire needling is a technique which involves quickly inserting a flame-heated needle into areas on the body.
- Sonopuncture is a stimulation of the body similar to acupuncture using sound instead of needles. This may be done using purpose-built transducers to direct a narrow ultrasound beam to a depth of 6–8 centimetres at acupuncture meridian points on the body. Alternatively, tuning forks or other sound emitting devices are used.
- Acupuncture point injection is the injection of various substances (such as drugs, vitamins or herbal extracts) into acupoints. This technique combines traditional acupuncture with injection of what is often an effective dose of an approved pharmaceutical drug, and proponents claim that it may be more effective than either treatment alone, especially for the treatment of some kinds of chronic pain. However, a 2016 review found that most published trials of the technique were of poor value due to methodology issues and larger trials would be needed to draw useful conclusions.
- Auriculotherapy, commonly known as ear acupuncture, auricular acupuncture, or auriculoacupuncture, is considered to date back to ancient China. It involves inserting needles to stimulate points on the outer ear. The modern approach was developed in France during the early 1950s. There is no scientific evidence that it can cure disease; the evidence of effectiveness is negligible.
- Scalp acupuncture, developed in Japan, is based on reflexological considerations regarding the scalp.
- Hand acupuncture, developed in Korea, centers around assumed reflex zones of the hand. Medical acupuncture attempts to integrate reflexological concepts, the trigger point model, and anatomical insights (such as dermatome distribution) into acupuncture practice, and emphasizes a more formulaic approach to acupuncture point location.
- Cosmetic acupuncture is the use of acupuncture in an attempt to reduce wrinkles on the face.
- Bee venom acupuncture is a treatment approach of injecting purified, diluted bee venom into acupoints.
- Veterinary acupuncture is the use of acupuncture on domesticated animals. Rigorous evidence for complementary and alternative techniques is lacking in veterinary medicine but evidence has been growing.

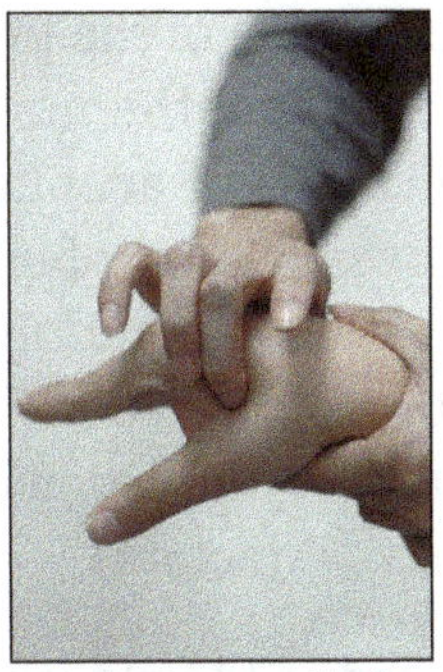

Acupressure being applied to a hand.

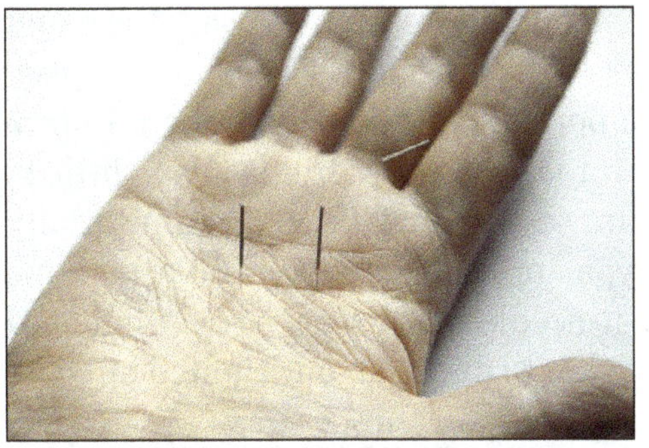

Sujichim, hand acupuncture.

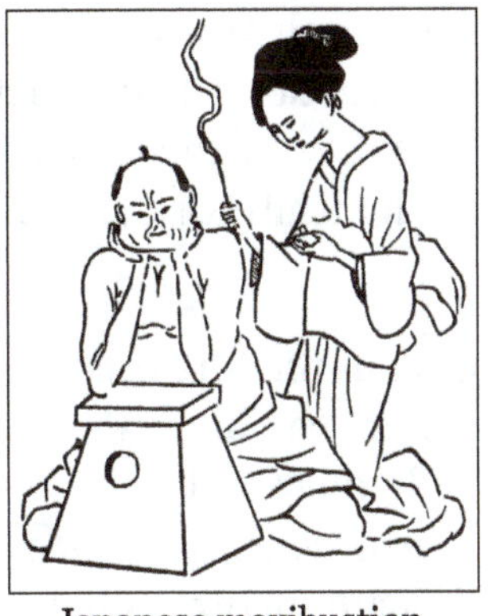

Japanese moxibustion.

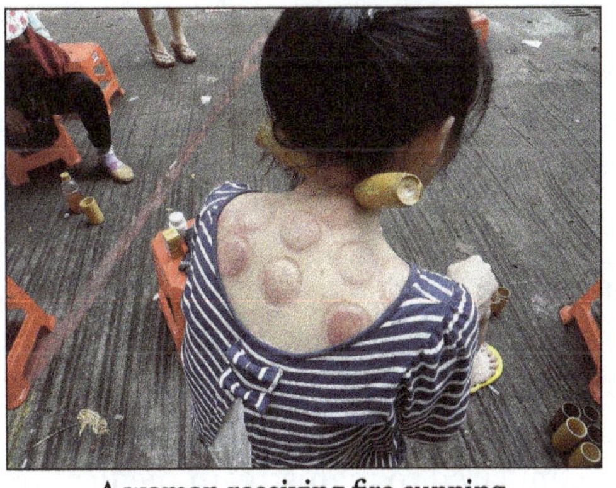

A woman receiving fire cupping.

Efficacy

Acupuncture has been researched extensively; as of 2013, there were almost 1,500 randomized controlled trials on PubMed with "acupuncture" in the title. The results of reviews of acupuncture's efficacy, however, have been inconclusive.

Sham Acupuncture and Research

It is difficult but not impossible to design rigorous research trials for acupuncture. Due to acupuncture's invasive nature, one of the major challenges in efficacy research is in the design of an appropriate placebo control group. For efficacy studies to determine whether acupuncture has specific effects, "sham" forms of acupuncture where the patient, practitioner, and analyst are blinded seem the most acceptable approach. Sham acupuncture uses non-penetrating needles or needling at non-acupuncture points, e.g. inserting needles on meridians not related to the specific condition being studied, or in places not associated with meridians. The under-performance of acupuncture in such trials may indicate that therapeutic effects are due entirely to non-specific effects, or that the sham treatments are not inert, or that systematic protocols yield less than optimal treatment.

A 2014 review found that "contrary to the claimed mechanism of redirecting the flow of *qi* through meridians, researchers usually find that it generally does not matter where the needles are inserted, how often (that is, no dose-response effect is observed), or even if needles are actually inserted. In other words, 'sham' or 'placebo' acupuncture generally produces the same effects as 'real' acupuncture and, in some cases, does better." A 2013 meta-analysis found little evidence that the effectiveness of acupuncture on pain (compared to sham) was modified by the location of the needles, the number of needles used, the experience or technique of the practitioner, or by the circumstances of the sessions. The same analysis also suggested that the number of needles and sessions is important, as greater numbers improved the outcomes of acupuncture compared to non-acupuncture controls. There has been little systematic investigation of which components of an acupuncture session may be important for any therapeutic effect, including needle placement and depth, type and intensity of stimulation, and number of needles used. The research seems to suggest that needles do not need to stimulate the traditionally specified acupuncture points or penetrate the skin to attain an anticipated effect (e.g. psychosocial factors).

A response to "sham" acupuncture in osteoarthritis may be used in the elderly, but placebos have usually been regarded as deception and thus unethical. However, some physicians and ethicists have suggested circumstances for applicable uses for placebos such as it might present a theoretical advantage of an inexpensive treatment without adverse reactions or interactions with drugs or other medications. As the evidence for most types of alternative medicine such as acupuncture is far from strong, the use of alternative medicine in regular healthcare can present an ethical question.

Using the principles of evidence-based medicine to research acupuncture is controversial, and has produced different results. Some research suggests acupuncture can alleviate pain but the majority of research suggests that acupuncture's effects are mainly due to placebo. Evidence suggests that any benefits of acupuncture are short-lasting. There is insufficient evidence to support use of acupuncture compared to mainstream medical treatments. Acupuncture is not better than mainstream treatment in the long term.

The use of acupuncture has been criticized owing to there being little scientific evidence for explicit effects, or the mechanisms for its supposed effectiveness, for any condition that is discernible from placebo. Acupuncture has been called 'theatrical placebo', and David Gorski argues that when acupuncture proponents advocate 'harnessing of placebo effects' or work on developing 'meaningful placebos', they essentially concede it is little more than that.

Specific Conditions

Pain

The conclusions of many trials and numerous systematic reviews of acupuncture are largely inconsistent with each other. A 2011 systematic review of systematic reviews found that for reducing pain, real acupuncture was no better than sham acupuncture, and concluded that numerous reviews have shown little convincing evidence that acupuncture is an effective treatment for reducing pain. The same review found that neck pain was one of only four types of pain for which a positive effect was suggested, but cautioned that the primary studies used carried a considerable risk of bias. A 2009 overview found acupuncture is not effective for a wide range of conditions.

A 2014 systematic review suggests that the nocebo effect of acupuncture is clinically relevant and that the rate of adverse events may be a gauge of the nocebo effect. A 2012 meta-analysis conducted by the Acupuncture Trialists' Collaboration found "relatively modest" efficacy of acupuncture (in comparison to sham) for the treatment of four different types of chronic pain (back and neck pain, knee osteoarthritis, chronic headache, and shoulder pain) and on that basis concluded that it "is more than a placebo" and a reasonable referral option. Commenting on this meta-analysis, both Edzard Ernst and David Colquhoun said the results were of negligible clinical significance. Edzard Ernst later stated that "I fear that, once we manage to eliminate this bias that operators are not blind we might find that the effects of acupuncture exclusively are a placebo response." In 2017, the same research group updated their previous meta-analysis and again found acupuncture to be superior to sham acupuncture for non-specific musculoskeletal pain, osteoarthritis, chronic headache, and shoulder pain. They also found that the effects of acupuncture decreased by about 15% after one year.

A 2010 systematic review suggested that acupuncture is more than a placebo for commonly occurring chronic pain conditions, but the authors acknowledged that it is still unknown if the overall benefit is clinically meaningful or cost-effective. A 2010 review found real acupuncture and sham acupuncture produce similar improvements, which can only be accepted as evidence against the efficacy of acupuncture. The same review found limited evidence that real acupuncture and sham acupuncture appear to produce biological differences despite similar effects. A 2009 systematic review and meta-analysis found that acupuncture had a small analgesic effect, which appeared to lack any clinical importance and could not be discerned from bias. The same review found that it remains unclear whether acupuncture reduces pain independent of a psychological impact of the needling ritual. A 2017 systematic review and meta-analysis found that ear acupuncture may be effective at reducing pain within 48 hours of its use, but the mean difference between the acupuncture and control groups was small.

Lower Back Pain

A 2013 systematic review found that acupuncture may be effective for nonspecific lower back pain, but the authors noted there were limitations in the studies examined, such as heterogeneity in study characteristics and low methodological quality in many studies. A 2012 systematic review found some supporting evidence that acupuncture was more effective than no treatment for chronic non-specific low back pain; the evidence was conflicting comparing the effectiveness over other treatment approaches. A 2011 systematic review of systematic reviews found that "for chronic low back pain, individualized acupuncture is not better in reducing symptoms than formula acupuncture or sham acupuncture with a toothpick that does not penetrate the skin." A 2010 review found that sham acupuncture was as effective as real acupuncture for chronic low back pain. The specific therapeutic effects of acupuncture were small, whereas its clinically relevant benefits were mostly due to contextual and psychosocial circumstances. Brain imaging studies have shown that traditional acupuncture and sham acupuncture differ in their effect on limbic structures, while at the same time showed equivalent analgesic effects. A 2005 Cochrane review found insufficient evidence to recommend for or against either acupuncture or dry needling for acute low back pain. The same review found low quality evidence for pain relief and improvement compared to no treatment or sham therapy for chronic low back pain only in the short term immediately after treatment. The same review also found that acupuncture is not more effective than conventional therapy and other alternative medicine treatments. A 2017 systematic review and meta-analysis concluded that, for neck pain, acupuncture was comparable in effectiveness to conventional treatment, while electroacupuncture was even more effective in reducing pain than was conventional acupuncture. The same review noted that "It is difficult to draw conclusion because the included studies have a high risk of bias and imprecision." A 2015 overview of systematic reviews of variable quality showed that acupuncture can provide short-term improvements to people with chronic low back pain. The overview said this was true when acupuncture was used either in isolation or in addition to conventional therapy. A 2017 systematic review for an American College of Physicians clinical practice guideline found low to moderate evidence that acupuncture was effective for chronic low back pain, and limited evidence that it was effective for acute low back pain. The same review found that the strength of the evidence for both conditions was low to moderate. Another 2017 clinical practice guideline, this one produced by the Danish Health Authority, recommended against acupuncture for both recent-onset low back pain and lumbar radiculopathy.

Headaches and Migraines

Two separate 2016 Cochrane reviews found that acupuncture could be useful in the prophylaxis of tension-type headaches and episodic migraines. The 2016 Cochrane review evaluating acupuncture for episodic migraine prevention concluded that true acupuncture had a small effect beyond sham acupuncture and found moderate-quality evidence to suggest that acupuncture is at least similarly effective to prophylactic medications for this purpose. A 2012 review found that acupuncture has demonstrated benefit for the treatment of headaches, but that safety needed to be more fully documented in order to make any strong recommendations in support of its use.

Arthritis Pain

A 2014 review concluded that "current evidence supports the use of acupuncture as an alternative to traditional analgesics in osteoarthritis patients." As of 2014, a meta-analysis showed that acupuncture may help osteoarthritis pain but it was noted that the effects were insignificant in comparison to sham needles. A 2012 review found "the potential beneficial action of acupuncture on osteoarthritis pain does not appear to be clinically relevant." A 2010 Cochrane review found that acupuncture shows statistically significant benefit over sham acupuncture in the treatment of peripheral joint osteoarthritis; however, these benefits were found to be so small that their clinical significance was doubtful, and "probably due at least partially to placebo effects from incomplete blinding".

A 2013 Cochrane review found low to moderate evidence that acupuncture improves pain and stiffness in treating people with fibromyalgia compared with no treatment and standard care. A 2012 review found "there is insufficient evidence to recommend acupuncture for the treatment of fibromyalgia." A 2010 systematic review found a small pain relief effect that was not apparently discernible from bias; acupuncture is not a recommendable treatment for the management of fibromyalgia on the basis of this review.

A 2012 review found that the effectiveness of acupuncture to treat rheumatoid arthritis is "sparse and inconclusive." A 2005 Cochrane review concluded that acupuncture use to treat rheumatoid arthritis "has no effect on ESR, CRP, pain, patient's global assessment, number of swollen joints, number of tender joints, general health, disease activity and reduction of analgesics." A 2010 overview of systematic reviews found insufficient evidence to recommend acupuncture in the treatment of most rheumatic conditions, with the exceptions of osteoarthritis, low back pain, and lateral elbow pain. A 2018 systematic review found some evidence that acupuncture could be effective for the treatment of rheumatoid arthritis, but that the evidence was limited because of heterogeneity and methodological flaws in the included studies.

Other Joint Pain

A 2014 systematic review found that although manual acupuncture was effective at relieving short-term pain when used to treat tennis elbow, its long-term effect in relieving pain was "unremarkable". A 2007 review found that acupuncture was significantly better than sham acupuncture at treating chronic knee pain; the evidence was not conclusive due to the lack of large, high-quality trials.

Post-operative Pain and Nausea

A 2014 overview of systematic reviews found insufficient evidence to suggest that acupuncture is an effective treatment for postoperative nausea and vomiting (PONV) in a clinical setting. A 2013 systematic review concluded that acupuncture might be beneficial in prevention and treatment of PONV. A 2015 Cochrane review found moderate-quality evidence of no difference between stimulation of the P6 acupoint on the wrist and antiemetic drugs for preventing PONV. A new finding of the review was that further comparative trials are futile, based on the conclusions of a trial sequential analysis. Whether combining PC6 acupoint stimulation with antiemetics is effective was inconclusive.

A 2014 overview of systematic reviews found insufficient evidence to suggest that acupuncture is effective for surgical or post-operative pain. For the use of acupuncture for post-operative pain, there was contradictory evidence. A 2014 systematic review found supportive but limited evidence for use of acupuncture for acute post-operative pain after back surgery. A 2014 systematic review found that while the evidence suggested acupuncture could be an effective treatment for postoperative gastroparesis, a firm conclusion could not be reached because the trials examined were of low quality.

Pain and Nausea Associated with Cancer and Cancer Treatment

A 2015 Cochrane review found that there is insufficient evidence to determine whether acupuncture is an effective treatment for cancer pain in adults. A 2014 systematic report, found that acupuncture may be effective as an adjunctive treatment to palliative care for cancer patients. A 2013 overview of report, found evidence that acupuncture could be beneficial for people with cancer-related symptoms, but also identified few rigorous trials and high heterogeneity between trials. A 2012 systematic report of randomised clinical trials, found that the number and quality of RCTs for using acupuncture in the treatment of cancer pain was too low to draw definite conclusions.

A 2014 systematic review reached inconclusive results with regard to the effectiveness of acupuncture for treating cancer-related fatigue. A 2013 systematic review found that acupuncture is an acceptable adjunctive treatment for chemotherapy-induced nausea and vomiting, but that further research with a low risk of bias is needed. A 2013 systematic review found that the quantity and quality of available RCTs for analysis were too low to draw valid conclusions for the effectiveness of acupuncture for cancer-related fatigue.

Sleep

A 2016 systematic review and meta-analysis found that acupuncture was "associated with a significant reduction in sleep disturbances in women experiencing menopause-related sleep disturbances."

Moxibustion and Cupping

A 2010 overview of systematic reviews found that moxibustion was effective for several conditions but the primary studies were of poor quality, so there persists ample uncertainty, which limits the conclusiveness of their findings.

Safety

Adverse Events

Acupuncture is generally safe when administered by an experienced, appropriately trained practitioner using clean-needle technique and sterile single-use needles. When improperly delivered it can cause adverse effects. Accidents and infections are associated with infractions of sterile technique or neglect on the part of the practitioner. To reduce the risk of serious adverse events after acupuncture, acupuncturists should be trained sufficiently. People with serious spinal disease, such as cancer or infection, are not good candidates for acupuncture. Contraindications to acupuncture (conditions that should not be treated with acupuncture) include coagulopathy disorders (e.g. hemophilia and advanced liver disease), warfarin use, severe psychiatric disorders (e.g. psychosis), and skin infections or skin trauma (e.g. burns). Further, electroacupuncture should be avoided at the spot of implanted electrical devices (such as pacemakers).

A 2011 systematic review of systematic reviews (internationally and without language restrictions) found that serious complications following acupuncture continue to be reported. Between 2000 and 2009, ninety-five cases of serious adverse events, including five deaths, were reported. Many such events are not inherent to acupuncture but are due to malpractice of acupuncturists. This might be why such complications have not been reported in surveys of adequately trained acupuncturists. Most such reports originate from Asia, which may reflect the large number of treatments performed there or a relatively higher number of poorly trained Asian acupuncturists. Many serious adverse events were reported from developed countries. These included Australia, Austria, Canada, Croatia, France, Germany, Ireland, the Netherlands, New Zealand, Spain, Sweden, Switzerland, the UK, and the US. The number of adverse effects reported from the UK appears particularly unusual, which may indicate less under-reporting in the UK than other countries. Reports included 38 cases of infections and 42 cases of organ trauma. The most frequent adverse events included pneumothorax, and bacterial and viral infections.

A 2013 review found (without restrictions regarding publication date, study type or language) 295 cases of infections; mycobacterium was the pathogen in at least 96%. Likely sources of infection include towels, hot packs or boiling tank water, and reusing reprocessed needles. Possible sources of infection include contaminated needles, reusing personal needles, a person's skin containing mycobacterium, and reusing needles at various sites in the same person. Although acupuncture is generally considered a safe procedure, a 2013 review stated that the reports of infection transmission increased significantly in the prior decade, including those of mycobacterium. Although it is recommended that practitioners of acupuncture use disposable needles, the reuse of sterilized needles is still permitted. It is also recommended that thorough control practices for preventing infection be implemented and adapted.

Children and Pregnancy

Although acupuncture has been practiced for thousands of years, its use in pediatrics in the United States did not become common until the early 2000s. In 2007, the National Health Interview Survey (NHIS) conducted by the National Center For Health Statistics (NCHS) estimated that approximately 150,000 children had received acupuncture treatment for a variety of conditions.

In 2008 a study determined that the use of acupuncture-needle treatment on children was "questionable" due to the possibility of adverse side-effects and the pain manifestation differences in children versus adults. The study also includes warnings against practicing acupuncture on infants, as well as on children who are over-fatigued, very weak, or have over-eaten.

When used on children, acupuncture is considered safe when administered by well-trained, licensed practitioners using sterile needles; however, a 2011 review found there was limited research to draw definite conclusions about the overall safety of pediatric acupuncture. The same review found 279 adverse events, 25 of them serious. The adverse events were mostly mild in nature (e.g. bruising or bleeding). The prevalence of mild adverse events ranged from 10.1% to 13.5%, an estimated 168 incidences among 1,422 patients. On rare occasions adverse events were serious (e.g. cardiac rupture or hemoptysis); many might have been a result of substandard practice. The incidence of serious adverse events was 5 per one million, which included children and adults.

When used during pregnancy, the majority of adverse events caused by acupuncture were mild and transient, with few serious adverse events. The most frequent mild adverse event was needling or unspecified pain, followed by bleeding. Although two deaths (one stillbirth and one neonatal death) were reported, there was a lack of acupuncture-associated maternal mortality. Limiting the evidence as certain, probable or possible in the causality evaluation, the estimated incidence of adverse events following acupuncture in pregnant women was 131 per 10,000. Although acupuncture is not contraindicated in pregnant women, some specific acupuncture points are particularly sensitive to needle insertion; these spots, as well as the abdominal region, should be avoided during pregnancy.

Moxibustion and Cupping

Four adverse events associated with moxibustion were bruising, burns and cellulitis, spinal epidural abscess, and large superficial basal cell carcinoma. Ten adverse events were associated with cupping. The minor ones were keloid scarring, burns, and bullae; the serious ones were acquired hemophilia A, stroke following cupping on the back and neck, factitious panniculitis, reversible cardiac hypertrophy, and iron deficiency anemia.

Cost-effectiveness

A 2013 meta-analysis found that acupuncture for chronic low back pain was cost-effective as a complement to standard care, but not as a substitute for standard care except in cases where comorbid depression presented. The same meta-analysis found there was no difference between sham and non-sham acupuncture. A 2011 systematic review found insufficient evidence for the cost-effectiveness of acupuncture in the treatment of chronic low back pain. A 2010 systematic review found that the cost-effectiveness of acupuncture could not be concluded. A 2012 review found that acupuncture seems to be cost-effective for some pain conditions.

Risk of Forgoing Conventional Medical Care

As with other alternative medicines, unethical or naïve practitioners may induce patients to exhaust financial resources by pursuing ineffective treatment. Professional ethics codes set by accrediting organizations such as the National Certification Commission for Acupuncture and Oriental Medicine require practitioners to make "timely referrals to other health care professionals as may be appropriate." Stephen Barrett states that there is a "risk that an acupuncturist whose approach to diagnosis is not based on scientific concepts will fail to diagnose a dangerous condition".

Conceptual Basis

Traditional

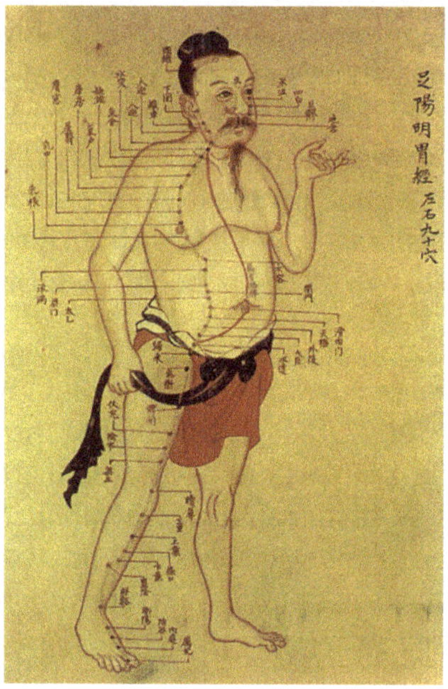

Old Chinese medical chart of acupuncture meridians.

Acupuncture is a substantial part of traditional Chinese medicine (TCM). Early acupuncture beliefs relied on concepts that are common in TCM, such as a life force energy called *qi*. *Qi* was believed to flow from the body's primary organs (zang-fu organs) to the "superficial" body tissues of the skin, muscles, tendons, bones, and joints, through channels called meridians. Acupuncture points where needles are inserted are mainly (but not always) found at locations along the meridians. Acupuncture points not found along a meridian are called extraordinary points and those with no designated site are called "A-shi" points.

In TCM, disease is generally perceived as a disharmony or imbalance in energies such as yin, yang, *qi*, xuě, zàng-fǔ, meridians, and of the interaction between the body and the environment. Therapy is based on which "pattern of disharmony" can be identified. For example, some diseases are believed to be caused by meridians being invaded with an excess of wind, cold, and damp. In order to determine which pattern is at hand, practitioners examine things like the color and shape of the tongue, the relative strength of pulse-points, the smell of the breath, the quality of breathing, or the sound of the voice. TCM and its concept of disease does not strongly differentiate between the cause and effect of symptoms.

Purported Scientific Basis

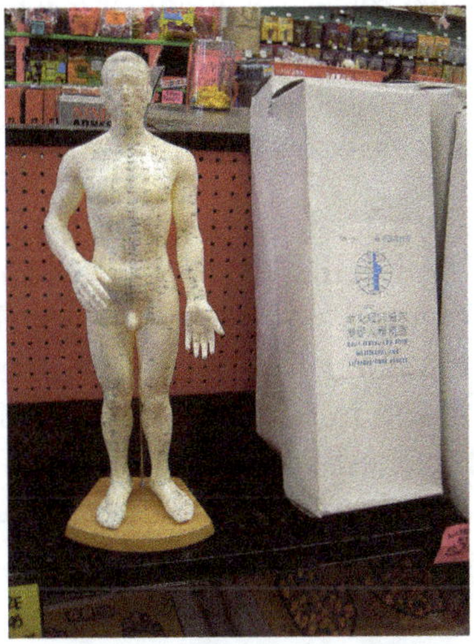

Modern acupuncture model.

Scientific research has not supported the existence of *qi*, meridians, or yin and yang. A *Nature* editorial described TCM as "fraught with pseudoscience", with the majority of its treatments having no logical mechanism of action. Quackwatch states that "TCM theory and practice are not based upon the body of knowledge related to health, disease, and health care that has been widely accepted by the scientific community. TCM practitioners disagree among themselves about how to diagnose patients and which treatments should go with which diagnoses. Even if they could agree, the TCM theories are so nebulous that no amount of scientific study will enable TCM to offer rational care."

Some modern practitioners support the use of acupuncture to treat pain, but have abandoned the use of qi, meridians, yin, yang and other mystical energies as an explanatory frameworks. The use of qi as an explanatory framework has been decreasing, even as it becomes more prominent during discussions of acupuncture in the US. Academic discussions of acupuncture still make reference to pseudoscientific concepts such as qi and meridians despite the lack of scientific evidence. Many within the scientific community consider attempts to rationalize acupuncture in science to be quackery and pseudoscience. Academics Massimo Pigliucci and Maarten Boudry describe it as a "borderlands science" lying between science and pseudoscience.

Many acupuncturists attribute pain relief to the release of endorphins when needles penetrate, but no longer support the idea that acupuncture can affect a disease. It is a generally held belief within the acupuncture community that acupuncture points and meridians structures are special conduits for electrical signals, but no research has established any consistent anatomical structure or function for either acupuncture points or meridians. Human tests to determine whether electrical continuity was significantly different near meridians than other places in the body have been inconclusive.

Some studies suggest acupuncture causes a series of events within the central nervous system, and that it is possible to inhibit acupuncture's analgesic effects with the opioid antagonist naloxone. Mechanical deformation of the skin by acupuncture needles appears to result in the release of adenosine. The anti-nociceptive effect of acupuncture may be mediated by the adenosine A1 receptor.

A 2014 review in Nature Reviews Cancer found that since the key mouse studies that suggested acupuncture relieves pain via the local release of adenosine, which then triggered nearby A1 receptors "caused more tissue damage and inflammation relative to the size of the animal in mice than in humans, such studies unnecessarily muddled a finding that local inflammation can result in the local release of adenosine with analgesic effect."

It has been proposed that acupuncture's effects in gastrointestinal disorders may relate to its effects on the parasympathetic and sympathetic nervous system, which have been said to be the "Western medicine" equivalent of "yin and yang". Another mechanism whereby acupuncture may be effective for gastrointestinal dysfunction involves the promotion of gastric peristalsis in subjects with low initial gastric motility, and suppressing peristalsis in subjects with active initial motility. Acupuncture has also been found to exert anti-inflammatory effects, which may be mediated by the activation of the vagus nerve and deactivation of inflammatory macrophages. Neuroimaging studies suggest that acupuncture stimulation results in deactivation of the limbic brain areas and the default mode network.

Adoption

Acupuncture is most heavily practiced and is popular in the US, Australia, and Europe. In Switzerland, acupuncture has become the most frequently used alternative medicine since 2004. In the United Kingdom, a total of 4 million acupuncture treatments were administered in 2009. Acupuncture is used in most pain clinics and hospices in the UK. An estimated 1 in 10 adults in Australia used acupuncture in 2004. In Japan, it is estimated that 25 percent of the population will try acupuncture at some point, though in most cases it is not covered by public health insurance. Users of acupuncture in Japan are more likely to be elderly and to have a limited education. Approximately half of users surveyed indicated a likelihood to seek such remedies in the future, while 37% did not. Less than one percent of the US population reported having used acupuncture in the early 1990s. By the early 2010s, more than 14 million Americans reported having used acupuncture as part of their health care.

In the US, acupuncture is increasingly (as of 2014) used at academic medical centers, and is usually offered through CAM centers or anesthesia and pain management services.

The use of acupuncture in Germany increased by 20% in 2007, after the German acupuncture trials supported its efficacy for certain uses. In 2011, there were more than one million users, and insurance companies have estimated that two-thirds of German users are women. As a result of the trials, German public health insurers began to cover acupuncture for chronic low back pain and osteoarthritis of the knee, but not tension headache or migraine. This decision was based in part on socio-political reasons. Some insurers in Germany chose to stop reimbursement of acupuncture because of the trials. For other conditions, insurers in Germany were not convinced that acupuncture had adequate benefits over usual care or sham treatments. Highlighting the results of the placebo group, researchers refused to accept a placebo therapy as efficient.

Acupuncture in Cardiology

Scientific studies using modern technology on acupuncture actually began in the late 1950s with further progress being made since the discovery of endogenous opioids in 1975. Much more advances have been made in more recent years in further understanding of the basic mechanisms underlying this millennium old medical treatment and its various clinical applications in the 21st century.

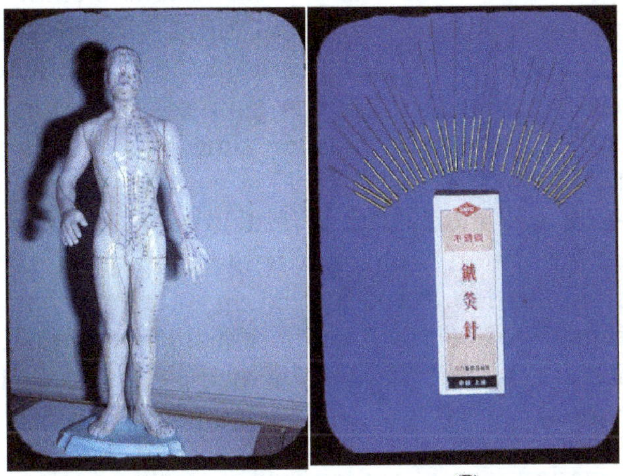

(A) (B)

(A)An acupuncture manikin showing the location of the various acupoints along the meridians; (B) a complete set of acupuncture needles.

Hypercholesterolemia

Electro-acupuncture has some therapeutic effect on decreasing the content of total cholesterol and low-density-lipoprotein cholesterol in hyperlipidemic rats and improving the gene expression of ATP-binding cassette transporter A1, peroxisome proliferator-activated receptor alpha, liver X receptor alpha and retinoid X receptor-alpha mRNA, so as to promote reverse cholesterol transport. Furthermore, real-time PCR and western blot indicate that electroacupuncture at ST 40 induces the expression of nNOS and Mt1, two genes involved in no signal transduction. Acupuncture treatment for hypercholesterolemia thus involves the modulation of several biological pathways and provides a physiological link between no signal transduction and the cholesterol-lowering effect of acupuncture.

Coronary Artery Disease

The effectiveness of acupuncture in treatment of angina has been well documented. Its antianginal effect has been shown to be secondary to an antiischemic effect, which in turn is due to a decrease in heart rate and blood pressure and reduction in left ventricular afterload, a reduction in myocardial oxygen consumption, and a redistribution of coronary blood flow, myocardial release of β-endorphin, coronary vasodilatation, and increase in coronary collateral circulation. Acupoint pressing has been shown to alleviate angina faster (2.45 +/- 1.67 min) than sublingual nitroglycerin (2.89 +/- 2.64 min). Transmyocardial acupuncture has also been used as a novel approach to myocardial revascularization, although its rationale has been questioned.

Acupuncture has been successfully used to improve microcirculation and left ventricular function in acute myocardial infarction. Animal studies demonstrated that electro-acupuncture could decrease the ST-segment elevation in ECG and reduce the infarct size following coronary ligation, although a recent study on rats failed to show a cardioprotective effect of electroacupuncture in terms of reduction of either infarct size or ventricular arrhythmias. Acupuncture has also been successfully employed to terminate nausea and vomiting and intractable hiccup complicating acute myocardial infarction.

Cardiac Arrhythmias

Acupuncture has been employed to treat both experimental and clinical arrhythmias. The latter included ventricular extrasystoles, sinus bradycardia, atrial fibrillation, decreased heart rate variability and sudden death. In the treatment of paroxysmal atrial fibrillation and atrial flutter, acupuncture at Neiguan, Shenmen, and Danzhong is more effective than intravenous amiodarone (conversion rate: 85% vs 67%, $p<0.01$; conversion time: 39.6+/-13.7 min vs 50.1+/-14.8 min, $p<0.01$). Acupuncture at Neiguan, Shenmen and Xinshu also can prevent recurrences of atrial fibrillation after cardioversion in patients with persistent atrial fibrillation. The advantage of acupuncture in treating atrial fibrillation is obvious, because it does not have any of the untoward effect of pharmacotherapy or ablation. Atrial fibrillation is the most common cardiac arrhythmia, and anxiety plays a significant role in either its initiation or its perpetuation. Because acupuncture is very effective in treating anxiety, this therapeutic modality warrants further investigation as a promising therapeutic option.

A recently published systematic review of randomized controlled trials failed to provide conclusive evidence in support of acupuncture treatment for cardiac arrhythmias. Furthermore, electro-acupuncture may interfere with demand pacemakers, although one recent case report from Greece indicated its safety. Electo-acupuncture may also trigger inappropriate ICD discharges. Therefore, extreme caution should be employed when electro-acupuncture is prescribed for patients with pacemakers and/or ICDs, and each patient should be considered individually with great care.

Congestive Heart Failure

In a Chinese echocardiographic study of patients with congestive heart failure due to dilated cardiomyopathy under maintenance doses of conventional drugs, including digitalis, diuretics and potassium supplements, acupuncture resulted in an increase in stroke volume. Because patients with heart failure have increased sympathetic activity and acupuncture produces release of endogenous opioids in the central nervous system which would inhibit central sympathetic outflow, sympathetic activation during acute mental stress was markedly attenuated or virtually eliminated after acupuncture. This may explain why ear acupuncture has been used in treating chronic heart failure, because one of the acupuncture points stimulated by the needle in the ear corresponds to the closest position of the vagus nerve to the cutaneous surface (vide infra), and electrical vagus nerve stimulation has been advocated for patients with advanced heart failure.

Acupuncture may become an additional therapeutic strategy to improve the exercise tolerance of patients with chronic heart failure, potentially by improving skeletal muscle function. The German researchers found a remarkable increase in 6-minute walk distance, improvement in ventilatory efficiency and post-exercise recovery, and increase in heart rate variability, despite a lack of improvement of the cardiac ejection fraction and peak oxygen uptake. They recommended that further research be carried out to understand the beneficial mechanisms of acupuncture in particular, its effects on neurohormonal balance and production of inflammatory cytokines.

In patients with chronic heart failure, acupuncture may reduce digitoxicity by regulating intracellular Ca^{++}, improving the function of Ca^{++}-ATPase in the sarcoplasmic reticulum, and increasing the calcium sensitivity of cardiac troponin. These considerations may provide a novel clue for attenuating the toxicity of digitalis preparations given to patients with chronic heart failure.

Hypertension

Experimental studies have shown that acupuncture inhibits the reflex-induced hypertension by modulating the activity of cardiovascular parasympathetic neurons in the rostral ventrolateral medulla. Activation of neurons in the arcuate nucleus of the hypothalamus, ventrolateral periaqueductal gray in the midbrain, and medullary nucleus raphé pallidus in the medulla by acupuncture can inhibit the activity of premotor sympathetic neurons in the rostral ventrolateral medulla. Glutamate, acetylcholine, opioids, gamma-aminobutyric acid, nociceptin, serotonin, nitric oxide and endocannabinoids in the brain all appear to participate in the antihypertensive response of acupuncture. Other possible mechanisms include decreases in plasma renin, plasma neuropeptide Y, aldosterone and angiotensin II activity; increased excretion of sodium; changes in plasma norepinephrine, serotonin and endorphin levels; and lowering of blood viscosity.

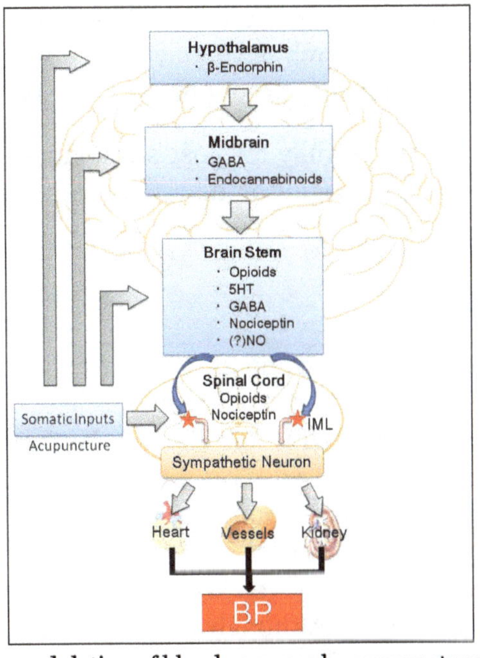

Neuroendocrine modulation of blood pressure by acupuncture. Abbreviations: GABA, γ-aminobutyric acid; 5HT, 5-hydroxytryptamine or serotonin; NO, nitric oxide; IML, intermediolateral column of the spinal cord.

However, the Stop Hypertension with the Acupuncture Research Program (SHARP) pilot trial concluded that acupuncture provided no greater benefit than invasive sham acupuncture in controlling moderate hypertension. Further research is obviously required to determine whether acupuncture can enhance clinical management of hypertension if used in combination with antihypertensive agents, over longer periods, or among specific subgroups of patients.

Stroke

Stroke should be considered as a coronary artery disease risk equivalent. Acupuncture has useful applications in both the acute and chronic phases of a stroke. In ischemic stroke, acupuncture increases local cerebral blood flow as determined by single photon emission computed tomography and near-infrared spectroscopy. In rats with ischemic stroke, acupuncture has been shown to promote angiogenesis. Acupuncture at Baihui and Fengchi is more effective than nimopidine in relieving cerebral vasospasm after embolization of ruptured aneurysms in subarachnoid hemorrhage. In a recent publication, the authors reviewed the progress of researches on the mechanism of acupuncture underlying improvement of acute cerebral hemorrhage from experimental studies and research methods. The effects of acupuncture mainly involve (1) lessening inflammatory reactions, (2) reducing impairment of free radicals and excitatory amino acids on cerebral neurons, (3) balancing release of vascular bioactive substances to increase regional cerebral blood flow, and (4) promoting repair and regeneration of the neural tissue. In regard to the research methods, many new biological techniques such as biological molecular approaches, neuro-cellular chemical methods, reverse transcription-polymerase chain reaction (RT-PCR) or quantitative real-time PCR, situ hybridization, western blotting, and electron microscopy have been extensively applied to researches on the underlying mechanisms of acupuncture therapy for cerebral infarction. In addition, the authors also pointed out that, in spite of achieving some greater progresses in experimental studies, most of the results basically reflect static, isolated and regional changes rather than dynamic and whole body changes. For these reasons, the authors recommended more in vivo research techniques and noninvasive research methods in the investigation of the underlying mechanisms of acupuncture therapy for acute cerebral ischemia.

Acupuncture has also been used successfully for post-stroke motor rehabilitation, behavioral recovery, aphasia, dysphasia, dysphagia, cognition disorders, depression, and urinary incontinence and urinary tract infection.

Smoking Cessation

Cigarette smoking is prevalent ; 67% of men and 40% of male physicians are smokers. It is a major cause of death and a principal cause of coronary heart disease. In addition, secondhand smoke exposure (52% of nonsmokers are exposed to tobacco smoke for at least 15 minutes daily for >1 day per week) was responsible for increased mortality due to coronary heart disease, ischemic stroke, lung cancer and chronic obstructive pulmonary disease in a recently published 17-year cohort study. Another recently completed Chinese population study, the Kailuan community study, showed smoking cessation to be one of the seven key components of an essential population-wide strategy to reduce cardiovascular disease. Although a 2012-15 blueprint on chronic disease prevention and control released by the Chinese Ministry of Health on May 21, 2012 set goals of reducing the adult smoking rate to below 25% among other goals, I have serious doubts as to how successful the Chinese Health Ministry's effort will be. Nevertheless, any effective measure in curtailing cigarette smoking should be actively and urgently pursued.

Acupuncture has been found in a recently published review of smoking cessation intervention studies to yield a much higher abstinence rate than pharmacotherapy or counseling. This observation was confirmed by two recently published meta-analyses of randomized controlled trials. It has been postulated that, by increasing the levels of endorphin, enkephalin, epinephrine, norepinephrine, serotonin, and dopamine in the central nervous system and plasma, acupuncture provides the smoker with a deterioration in the taste of smoking, a decrease in the desire of smoking, and the obstruction of psychological symptoms resulting from smoking cessation. The latest theory is that one of the acupuncture points stimulated by the acupuncture needle in the ear corresponds to the closest position of the vagus nerve to the cutaneous surface. Therefore, by stimulating this point, the acupuncturist blocks the outflow of withdrawal symptoms coming from the parasympathetic nervous system through the vagus nerve. However, more studies are needed to determine whether acupuncture is as efficacious as, or even more so than, pharmacotherapies.

Diabetes

Diabetes is associated with a marked increase in the risk of coronary artery disease, so much so that patients with diabetes shuld be treated as if they have existing coronary artery disease. As a matter of fact, diabetes should be considered as a coronary artery disease equivalent. The prevalence of diabetes is rising. The main reasons for the rising prevalence of diabetes are smoking and obesity, which are certainly true for China.

On the other hand, acupuncture has been found to be effective in the management of patients with diabetes, by causing the release of endogenous opioid peptides such as β-endorphin from adrenal gland and thereby enhancing insulin secretion. A recent literature review showed acupuncture to be effective in lowering blood glucose in both humans and rats. Ear acupuncture in 45 diabetics resulted in significant improvement in fasting plasma glucose, blood glucose load after 2-hour 75 gm oral glucose tolerance test and glycosylated hemoglobin. Two recent studies on patients with impaired glucose tolerance reported similar improvement in these parameters following electro-acupuncture, thus confirming its effectiveness in the prevention and treatment of diabetes at the early stage. Another study reported acupuncture to be effective in lowering fasting blood leptin level, which may contribute to its clinical effect in improving diabetes. Electro-acupuncture has also been used successfully for the treatment of diabetic peripheral neuropathy in rats as well as in patients, although the quality of reports about randomized controlled trials is moderate to low. Finally, acupuncture has been used in treating urinary tract infection in diabetic patients.

Obesity

Obesity is another risk factor for coronary artery disease, hypertension, chronic heart failure, stroke and diabetes. It is increasing in prevalence worldwide, especially in developing countries like China. Two recent systematic reviews, one published in 2009 and the other in 2012, both suggested that acupuncture is an effective treatment for obesity, with fewer adverse effects of the various dieting plans and Western anti-obesity drugs. A recent study in obese rats showed that electro-acupuncture led to a reduction of body weight, decrease in the plasma leptin levels, and an increase in leptin receptor expression in the hypothalamus, suggesting that regulating the expression of leptin and the leptin receptor might be one of the molecular mechanisms underlying the reduction of body weight in diet-induced obese rats by electro-acupuncture treatment. Another human study reported in 2010 found that laser acupuncture exerted a therapeutic effect on simple obesity by reducing both body weight and body mass index. However, the amount of evidence is not fully convincing, because of the small sample size and poor methodological quality of all the reported trials to date.

Adverse Effects and Complications

Although acupuncture is extremely safe, adverse effects and sometimes serious complications have been reported. These include infective endocarditis, pericardial effusion, cardiac tamponade, pneumothorax and AIDS. However, infective endocarditis and AIDS are not due to acupuncture per se, but to the unsterile technique that was employed during acupuncture. Hundreds of thousands of acupuncturists worldwide perform millions of acupuncture procedures per year. Considering the small number of reported complications in the literature, acupuncture is very safe indeed. As a matter of fact, the recent report of the successful use of electro-acupuncture for treatment of arthritis in a patient with a total artificial heart is further testimonial to its safety.

Acupuncture has a definite place in cardiology. When performed by trained acupuncturists, it is safe, effective, cost-effective, and widely available. As more research evidence for acupuncture efficacy, including the application of functional magnetic resonance imaging technique in recent years, becomes available, it will be possible to increase physician knowledge and change attitudes towards acupuncture

ANTHROPOSOPHICAL MEDICINE

Anthroposophic medicine (or anthroposophical medicine) is a form of alternative medicine. Devised in the 1920s by Rudolf Steiner in conjunction with Ita Wegman, anthroposophical medicine is based on occult notions and draws on Steiner's spiritual philosophy, which he called anthroposophy. Practitioners employ a variety of treatment techniques based upon anthroposophic precepts, including massage, exercise, counselling, and substances.

Many drug preparations used in anthroposophic medicine are ultra-diluted substances, similar to those used in homeopathy. Homeopathic remedies are not medically effective and are generally considered harmless, except when used as a substitute for a scientifically proven and effective cure. In certain European countries, people with cancer are sometimes prescribed remedies made from specially harvested mistletoe, but research has found no convincing evidence of clinical benefit. Some anthroposophic doctors oppose childhood vaccination, and this has led to preventable outbreaks of disease.

Anthroposophic medicine departs from fundamental biological principles in several respects. For example, Steiner said that the heart does not pump blood but that blood propels itself along. Anthroposophic medicine also proposes that patients' past lives may influence their illness and that the course of an illness is subject to karmic destiny. Professor of complementary medicine Edzard Ernst and other physicians and scientists including Simon Singh and David Gorski have characterized anthroposophic medicine as pseudoscientific quackery with no basis in reason or logic.

Co-founders of anthroposophic medicine

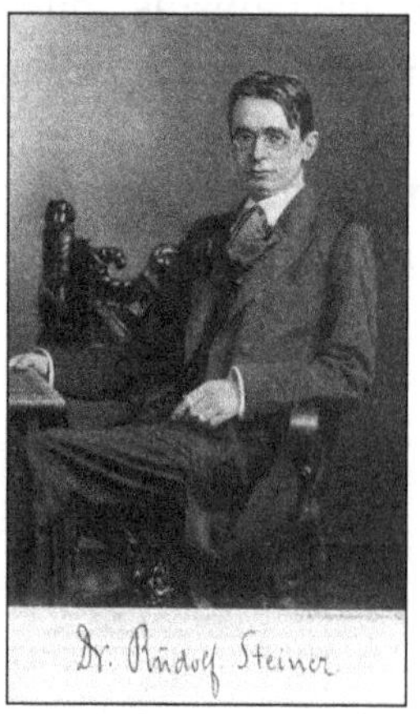

Rudolf Steiner.

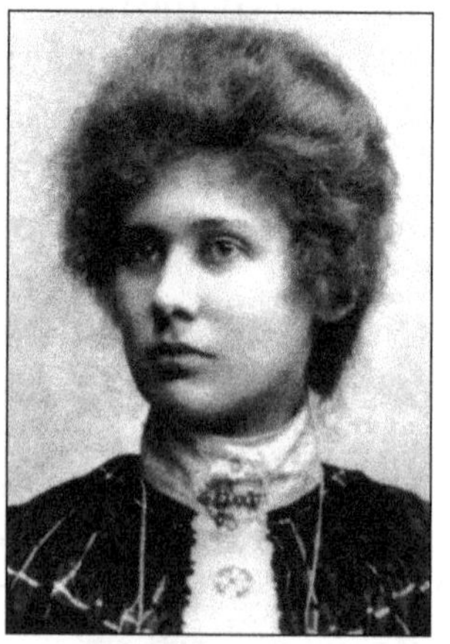

Ita Wegman.

The first steps towards an anthroposophic approach to medicine were made before 1920, when homeopathic physicians and pharmacists began working with Rudolf Steiner, who recommended new medicinal substances as well as specific methods for preparation along with an anthroposophic concept of man. In 1921, Ita Wegman opened the first anthroposophic medical clinic, now known as the Klinik Arlesheim, in Arlesheim, Switzerland. Wegman was soon joined by a number of other doctors. They then began to train the first anthroposophic nurses for the clinic.

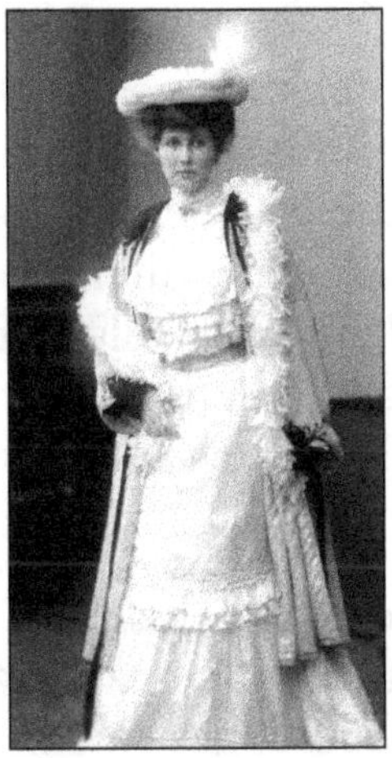

Ita Wegman, co-founder of the medical approach, before 1900 in Berlin.

At Wegman's request, Steiner regularly visited the clinic and suggested treatment regimes for particular patients. Between 1920 and 1925, he also gave several series of lectures on medicine. In 1925, Wegman and Steiner wrote the first book on the anthroposophic approach to medicine, Fundamentals of Therapy.

Wegman later opened a separate clinic and curative home in Ascona. Wegman lectured widely, visiting the Netherlands and England particularly frequently, and an increasing number of doctors began to include the anthroposophic approach in their practices. A cancer clinic, the Lukas Clinic, opened in Arlesheim in 1963.

In 1976 anthroposophic medicine in Germany got regulated by law as a specific therapeutic system by the Medicines Act-Arzneimittelgesetz (AMG) and by the Code of Social Law (Sozialgesetzbuch V).

In the 1990s the Witten/Herdecke University in Germany established a chair in anthroposophical medicine. The press described the appointment as a "death sentence" and the perception that pseudoscience was being taught damaged the university's reputation, bringing it close to financial collapse. It was ultimately saved by a cash injection from Software AG, a technology corporation with a history of funding anthroposophic projects.

In 2006, anthroposophical medicine was practised in 80 countries.

In 2012 the University of Aberdeen considered establishing a chair in holistic health jointly funded by Software AG, and by the Anthroposophic Health, Education, and Social Care Movement, each of which would provide £1.5 million of endowment. Edzard Ernst commented "that any decent university should even consider an anthroposophical medicine unit seems incomprehensible. The fact that it would be backed by people who have a financial interest in this bogus approach makes it even worse." The University's governance and nominations committee eventually decided not to proceed with the appointment.

Categorization and Conceptual Basis

The categorization of anthroposophical medicine is complex since in part it complements conventional medicine, and in part it substitutes for it. In 2008, Ernst wrote that it was being promoted as an "extension to conventional medicine".

Ernst writes that Steiner used imagination and insight as a basis for his ideas, drawing mystical knowledge from the occult Akashic Records, a work which is supposedly situated on the astral plane, and which Steiner said was accessible to him via his intuitive powers. On this basis, Steiner proposed "associations between four postulated dimensions of the human body (physical body, etheric body, astral body, and ego), plants, minerals, and the cosmos". Steiner also proposed a connection betweens planets, metals and organs so that, for example, the planet Mercury, the element mercury and the lung were all somehow associated. These propositions form the basis of anthroposophical medicine.

Ernst has said that anthroposophical medicine "includes some of the least plausible theories one could possibly imagine", categorized it as "pure quackery", and said that it "has no basis in science". According to Quackwatch, anthroposophical medicine practitioners regard illness as a "rite of passage" necessary to purge spiritual impurities carried over from past lives, according to the precepts of "karmic destiny".

Methods

In anthroposophic pharmacy drugs are prepared according to ancient notions of alchemy and homeopathy which are not related to the science underlying modern pharmacology. During the preparation process, patterns formed by crystallization are interpreted to see which "etheric force" they most closely resemble. Most anthroposophic preparations are highly diluted, like homeopathic remedies. This means that, while they are completely harmless in themselves, using them in place of conventional medicine to treat serious illness carries a risk of severe adverse consequences.

As well as drug remedies, anthroposophical medicine also includes:

- Anthroposophic nursing.
- Counselling.
- Eurythmy claimed to have an effect on "inner life functions" leading to a "re-integration of body, soul, and spirit".
- External applications.
- Rhythmic massages.

Plant-derived Treatments

To select an anthroposophic substance for a particular illness, practitioners consider the source of the substances used. The character of a mineral, plant or animal is hypothesised to have been formed by the substances that are most active within it, in the belief that this character may also influence what the substance will accomplish when given to treat another organism. This is related to Samuel Hahnemann's Doctrine of signatures. Willow, for example, is considered to have an unusual character:

> Plants that grow near water are usually heavy, with big, dark green leaves that wilt and break easily. An exception is the white willow, a tree that always grows near water and loves light. However, unlike other "watery" plants, the willow has fine, almost dry leaves and looks very light . Its branches are unbelievably tough. They are elastic and cannot be broken. They bend easily and form "joints" rather than break. These few signatures can give us the clue to what salix can be used for therapeutically: arthritis, deformation of joints, swollen joints.

There is no scientific evidence that the shape of plants has ever caused a new medical property to be discovered.

Beliefs about Human Biology

Steiner described the heart not as a pump, but as a regulator of flow, such that the heartbeat itself can be distinguished from the circulation of blood. Anthroposophic medicine claims the flow in the blood of the circulatory system is, as Marinelli put it, "propelled with its own biological momentum, as can be seen in the embryo, and boosts itself with induced momenta from the heart".

This view of the heart is not based on any scientific theory and has been characterized as "crank science".

Steiner believed that the sex of a baby was determined at the moment of conception by the alignment of the stars.

Steiner's model of anatomy was based on a three-part notion, whereby the head is the thinking part, the abdomen and limbs the "metabolic" part, and the chest and heart a "rhythmic center".

Mistletoe Treatment for Cancer

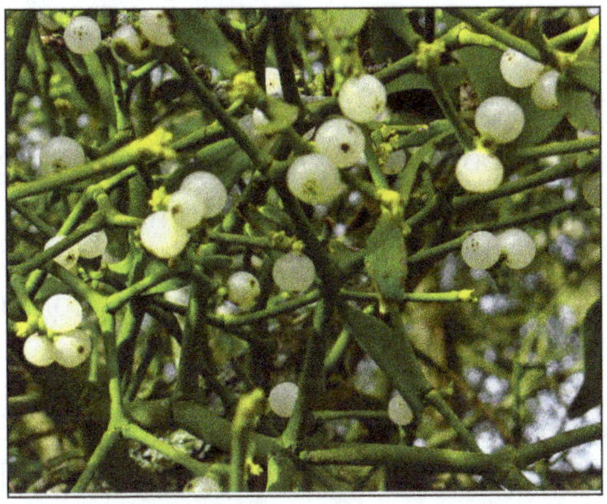

Mistletoe – Steiner said that harvesting it when the planets were aligned would yield a cancer treatment.

Rudolf Steiner hypothesised that mistletoe could cure cancer, on the basis of the observation that the plant was a parasite which eventually killed its host, a process which he claimed paralleled the progression of cancer. Steiner believed the plant's medical potential was influenced by the position of the sun, moon and planets and that it therefore was important to harvest the plant at the right time. Some mistletoe preparations are ultra-diluted; others are made from fermented mistletoe. The most commonly used trade names for mistletoe drugs are Iscador and Helixor.

Although laboratory experiments have suggested that mistletoe extract may affect the immune system and be able to kill some kinds of cancer cells, there is little evidence of its benefit to people with cancer. Most of the clinical research claiming that mistletoe therapy is effective is published in Germany, and it is generally considered unreliable because of major lapses in quality. Edzard Ernst wrote that research by anthroposophic doctors often reached positive conclusions on mistletoe therapy because it drew on unreliable material; independent researchers tended instead to find no evidence of benefit. The American Cancer Society says that "available evidence from well-designed clinical trials does not support claims that mistletoe can improve length or quality of life".

Mistletoe-based cancer drugs are widely used in Europe, especially in German-speaking countries. In 2002 nearly half a million prescriptions were paid for by German health insurance and in 2006 there were reportedly around 30 types of mistletoe extract on the market. Mistletoe extracts have been used as an unconventional treatment for cancer patients in the Netherlands, and in Germany the treatment has been approved as palliative therapy to treat the symptoms of patients with malignant tumors. In Sweden, controversially, mistletoe therapy has been approved for use in the treatment of cancer symptoms.

In other countries mistletoe therapy is virtually unknown. The United States Food and Drug Administration has not approved mistletoe-based drugs for any purpose; mistletoe extracts may not be distributed in or imported into the US except for research purposes. As of 2015 no mistletoe-based drugs are licensed for use in the United Kingdom.

A 2013 study on mistletoe in Lancet Oncology invoked Ben Goldacre's observation that a geographical preference for certain therapies was a hallmark of quackery, and proposed that the continuing use of this "apparently ineffectual therapy" in a small cluster of countries was based on sociological rather than medical reasons, indicating a need for a more informed consent from patients.

Immunization

The risks arising from using anthroposophical medicine as a substitute for evidence-based medicine are exemplified by several cases of low vaccination levels in Waldorf schools, since some anthroposophical doctors oppose immunization. A 1999 study of children in Sweden showed that in Waldorf schools, only 18% had received MMR vaccination, compared to a level of 93% in other schools nationally.

A 2003 report of a widespread measles outbreak around Coburg, Germany, identified a Waldorf school as the origin. At the time the town's mayor had condemned homeopathic doctors who had discouraged vaccination, saying "Their stronghold is the Waldorf School, which actively encourages people not to have their children vaccinated. Now we have an epidemic."

Paul Offit wrote that Steiner believed vaccination "interferes with karmic development and the cycles of reincarnation", and that adherence to this belief led to a 2008 pertussis outbreak in a Californian Waldorf school, causing its temporary closure.

APITHERAPY

Apitherapy is a branch of alternative medicine that uses honey bee products, including honey, pollen, propolis, royal jelly and bee venom. Proponents of apitherapy make claims for its health benefits which are unsupported by evidence-based medicine.

References to medical properties of bee products can be found in Chinese, Korean, Russian and Egyptian traditional medicine practices. Apitherapy has been practiced since the times of Hippocrates and Galen. The more modern study of apitherapy, specifically using bee venom, was initiated by Austrian physician Philipp Terč in his 1888 report "About a Peculiar Connection Between the Bee stings and Rheumatism." More recent alternative medicine practice is attributed to the Hungarian physician Bodog F. Beck who coined the term "bee venom therapy" in 1935, and to beekeeper Charles Mraz in the latter half of the twentieth century. In 1957, the USSR Ministry of Health sanctioned use of bee venom to treat certain ailments by approval of Nikolay Artemov's "Instruction for Bee Sting Venom Apitherapy."

Health Claims

Apitherapy is promoted as alternative medicine for several uses, but its health claims are not supported by scientific evidence. Bee venom or other honeybee products are ineffective for the treatment or prevention of cancer.

In general, evidence for using honey in wound treatment is of such low quality that firm conclusions cannot be drawn.

Risks

Adverse reactions to bee venom therapy are frequent. Frequent exposure to the venom can also lead to arthropathy. In sensitized persons, venom compounds can act as allergens, causing a spectrum of allergic reactions that can range from mild, local swelling to severe systemic reactions, anaphylactic shock, or even death.

In March 2018 it was reported that a 55-year-old woman died after receiving "live bee acupuncture", suffering a severe anaphylactic episode which the apitherapy practitioner did not respond to by administering adrenaline. While stabilized by ambulance personnel on the way to the hospital, she died a few weeks later from complications resulting in multiple organ failure. Live bee acupuncture therapy is "unsafe and unadvisable," according to researchers who studied the case.

HYPNOTHERAPY

Hypnotherapy is a form of complementary therapy that utilises the power of positive suggestion to bring about subconscious change to our thoughts, feelings and behaviour.

Hypnosis is thought to work by altering our state of consciousness in such a way that the analytical left-hand side of the brain is turned off, while the non-analytical right-hand side is made more alert. The conscious control of the mind is inhibited, and the subconscious mind awoken. Since the subconscious mind is a deeper-seated, more instinctive force than the conscious mind, this is the part which has to change for the patient's behaviour and physical state to alter.

Heading

Hypnotherapy is a talking therapy involving hypnosis which focuses a clients imagination and subconscious to help bring about positive changes to their thoughts, feelings or behaviour. Together the hypnotherapist and client will decide on the desired changes to work on prior to the hypnosis occurring.

Hypnotherapy is the use of different types of therapy in hypnosis, along with the mind's own natural abilities, to resolve issues, relieve emotional burdens and achieve personal goals. It is a safe, effective process and involves the client and therapist working together to bring about positive changes in how they think, feel and act.

Hypnotherapy is a kind of psychotherapy. Hypnotherapy aims to re-programme patterns of behaviour within the mind, enabling irrational fears, phobias, negative thoughts and suppressed emotions to be overcome. As the body is released from conscious control during the relaxed trance-like state of hypnosis, breathing becomes slower and deeper, the pulse rate drops and the metabolic rate falls.

Unlike counselling, psychotherapy or psychology which may involve looking at a number of issues in a conscious way, hypnotherapy often focuses on a singular issue and works with the unconscious. However this doesn't mean you risk losing control or that you can be manipulated to do or think things you don't want to. At all times when being hypnotised the client actually should remain in control and although very relaxed, should be able to talk or get up and leave the room if they want to.

Contrary to popular belief, hypnosis is not a state of deep sleep. It does involve the induction of a trance-like condition, but when in it, the patient is actually in an enhanced state of awareness, concentrating entirely on the hypnotist's voice. In this state, the conscious mind is suppressed and the subconscious mind is revealed.The therapist is able to suggest ideas, concepts and lifestyle adaptations to the patient, the seeds of which become firmly planted.

This method of hypnosis is not meant to cure or directly change a patient's behavior. It's meant to locate a cause and treat it through psychotherapy

What Issues is Hypnotherapy Suitable for Treating?

- Fears and Phobias (flying, public speaking etc).
- Weight Loss.
- Comfort Eating.
- Anxiety disorders, Panic Attacks.
- Insomnia and Sleeplessness.
- Obsessive Compulsive Disorder.

- Mild Depression.
- Habitual Behaviour (smoking, stammering,snoring,teeth grinding, sleepwalking, nail biting,bed wetting).
- Relationships.
- Allergies.
- Post traumatic stress disorder (PTSD).
- Pain management.
- Sexual problems.
- Confidence issues.
- Memory.

Types of Hypnotherapy

- Traditional/suggestion hypnotherapy.
- Analytical hypnotherapy/hypnoanalysis.
- Solution focused hypnotherapy.
- Hypno-psychotherapy.
- Clinical hypnotherapy.
- Cognitive/behavioural hypnotherapy.
- Hypnotherapy and NLP(Neuro-linguistic programming (NLP)).
- Time line therapy.

BATES METHOD

The Bates method is an ineffective alternative therapy aimed at improving eyesight. Eye-care physician William Horatio Bates, M.D. (1860–1931) attributed nearly all sight problems to habitual strain of the eyes, and felt that glasses were harmful and never necessary. Bates self-published a book, Perfect Sight Without Glasses, as well as a magazine, Better Eyesight Magazine, (and earlier collaborated with Bernarr MacFadden on a correspondence course) detailing his approach to helping people relax such "strain", and thus, he claimed, improve their sight. His techniques centered on visualization and movement. He placed particular emphasis on imagining black letters and marks, and the movement of such. He also proposed that exposing the eyes to sunlight would help alleviate the "strain".

Despite continued anecdotal reports of successful results, including well-publicised support by Aldous Huxley, Bates' techniques have not been objectively shown to improve eyesight. His main physiological proposition that the eyeball changes shape to maintain focus has consistently been contradicted by observation. In 1952, optometry professor Elwin Marg wrote of Bates, "Most of his claims and almost all of his theories have been considered false by practically all visual scientists." Marg concluded that the Bates method owed its popularity largely to "flashes of clear vision" experienced by many who followed it. Such occurrences have since been explained as a contact lens-like effect of moisture on the eye, or a flattening of the lens by the ciliary muscles.

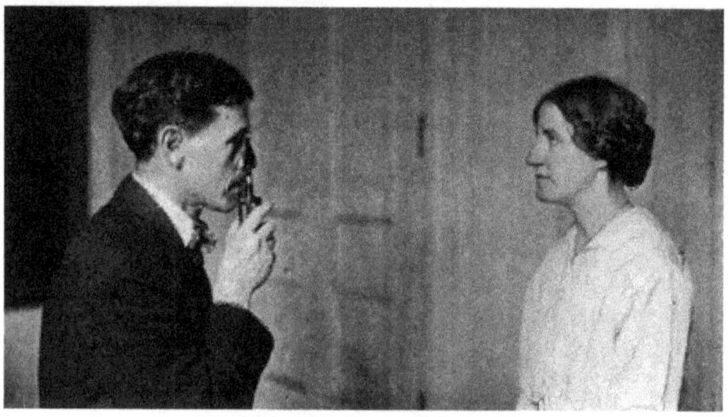

William Bates and his assistant.

The Bates method has been criticized not only because there is no good evidence it works, but also because it can have negative consequences for those who attempt to follow it: they might damage their eyes through overexposure of their eyes to sunlight, put themselves and others at risk by not wearing their corrective lenses while driving, or neglect conventional eye care, possibly allowing serious conditions to develop.

Underlying Concepts

Accommodation

Accommodation is the process by which the eye increases optical power to maintain focus on the retina while shifting its gaze to a closer point. The long-standing medical consensus is that this is accomplished by action of the ciliary muscle, a muscle within the eye, which adjusts the curvature of the eye's crystalline lens. This explanation is based in the observed effect of atropine temporarily preventing accommodation when applied to the ciliary muscle, as well as images reflected on the crystalline lens becoming smaller as the eye shifts focus to a closer point, indicating a change in the lens' shape. Bates rejected this explanation, and in his 1920 book presented photographs that he said showed that the image remained the same size even as the eye shifted focus, concluding from this that the lens was not a factor in accommodation. However, optometrist Philip Pollack in a 1956 work characterized these photographs as "so blurred that it is impossible to tell whether one image is larger than the other", in contrast to later photographs that clearly showed a change in the size of the reflected images, just as had been observed since the late 19th century.

Bates adhered to a different explanation of accommodation that had already been generally disregarded by the medical community of his time. Bates' model had the muscles surrounding the eyeball controlling its focus. In addition to their known function of turning the eye, Bates maintained, they also affect its shape, elongating the eyeball to focus at the near-point or shortening it to focus at a distance. Commenting on this hypothesis in an interview with WebMD, ophthalmologist Richard E. Bensinger stated, "When we put drops in the eye to dilate the pupil, they paralyze the focusing muscles. The evidence of the anatomical fallacy is that you can't focus, but your eye can move up and down, left and right. The notion that external muscles affect focusing is totally wrong." Science author John Grant writes that many animals, such as fishes, accommodate by elongation of the eyeball, "it's just that humans aren't one of those animals."

Laboratory tests have shown that the human eyeball is far too rigid to spontaneously change shape to a degree that would be necessary to accomplish what Bates described. Exceedingly small changes in axial length of the eyeball (18.6–19.2 μm) are caused by the action of the ciliary muscle during accommodation. However, these changes are far too small to account for the necessary changes in focus, producing changes of only −0.036 dioptres.

Causes of Sight Problems

Medical professionals characterize refractive errors such as nearsightedness, farsightedness, astigmatism, and presbyopia (the age-related blurring of near-point vision) as consequences of the eye's shape and other basic anatomy, for which no evidence shows that any exercise can alter. Bates, however, believed that these conditions are caused by tension of the muscles surrounding the eyeball, which he believed prevents the eyeball from sufficiently changing shape (per his explanation of accommodation) when gaze is shifted nearer or farther. Bates characterized this supposed muscular tension as the consequence of a "mental strain" to see, the relief of which he claimed would instantly improve sight. He also linked disturbances in the circulation of blood, which he said is "very largely influenced by thought", not only to refractive errors, but also to double vision, crossed-eye, lazy eye, and to more serious eye conditions such as cataracts and glaucoma. His therapies were based on these assumptions.

Bates felt that corrective lenses, which he characterized as "eye crutches", are an impediment to curing poor vision. In his view, "strain" would increase as the eyes adjust to the correction in front of them. He thus recommended that glasses be discarded by anyone applying his method.

Treatments

In his writings, Bates discussed several techniques that he claimed helped patients to improve their sight. He wrote "The ways in which people strain to see are infinite, and the methods used to relieve the strain must be almost equally varied," emphasizing that no single approach would work for everyone. His techniques were all designed to help disassociate this "strain" from seeing and thereby achieve "central fixation", or seeing what is in the central point of vision without staring. He asserted that "all errors of refraction and all functional disturbances of the eye disappear when it sees by central fixation" and that other conditions were often relieved as well.

Palming

Bates suggested closing the eyes for minutes at a time to help bring about relaxation. He asserted that the relaxation could be deepened in most cases by "palming", or covering the closed eyes with the palms of the hands, without putting pressure on the eyeballs. If the covered eyes did not strain, he said, they would see "a field so black that it is impossible to remember, imagine, or see anything blacker", since light was excluded by the palms. However, he reported that some of his patients experienced "illusions of lights and colors" sometimes amounting to "kaleidoscopic appearances" as they "palmed", occurrences he attributed to his ubiquitous "strain" and that he claimed disappeared when one truly relaxed. This phenomenon, however, was almost certainly caused by Eigengrau or "dark light". In fact, even in conditions of perfect darkness, as inside a cave, neurons at every level of the visual system produce random background activity that is interpreted by the brain as patterns of light and color.

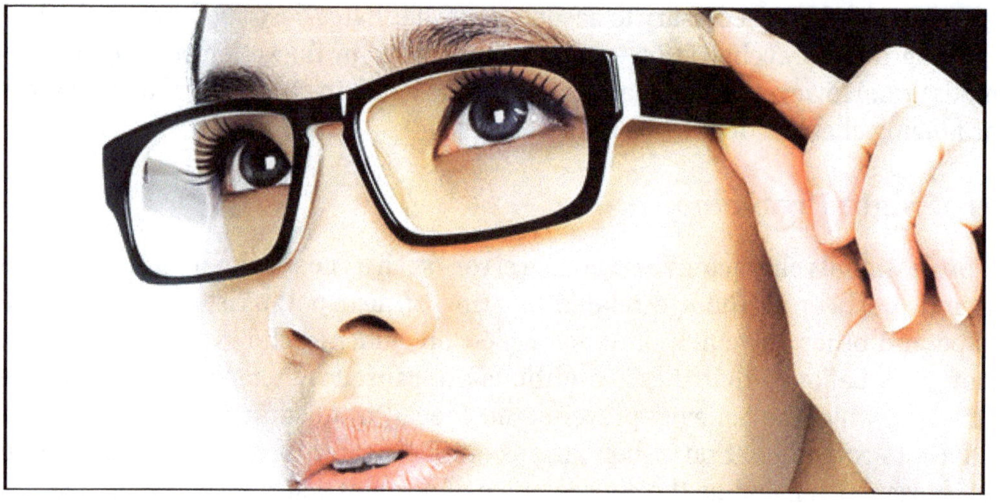

Visualization

Bates placed importance on mental images, as he felt relaxation was the key to clarity of imagination as well as of actual sight. He claimed that one's poise could be gauged by the visual memory of black; that the darker it appeared in the mind, and the smaller the area of black that could be imagined, the more relaxed one was at the moment. He recommended that patients think of the top letter from an eye chart and then visualize progressively smaller black letters, and eventually a period or comma, but he emphasized his view that the clear visual memory of black "cannot be attained by any sort of effort", stating that "the memory is not the cause of the relaxation, but must be preceded by it," and cautioned against "concentrating" on black, as he regarded an attempt to "think of one thing only" as a strain.

While Bates preferred to have patients imagine something black, he also reported that some found objects of other colors easiest to visualize, thus were benefited most by remembering those, because, he asserted, "the memory can never be perfect unless it is easy." Skeptics reason that the only benefit to eyesight gained from such techniques is itself imagined, and point out that familiar objects, including letters on an eye chart, can be recognized even when they appear less than clear.

Movement

He thought that the manner of eye movement affected the sight. He suggested "shifting", or moving the eyes back and forth to get an illusion of objects "swinging" in the opposite direction. He believed that the smaller the area over which the "swing" was experienced, the greater was the benefit to sight. He also indicated that it was usually helpful to close the eyes and imagine something "swinging". By alternating actual and mental shifting over an image, Bates wrote, many patients were quickly able to shorten the "shift" to a point where they could "conceive and swing a letter the size of a period in a newspaper". One who mastered this would attain the "universal swing", Bates believed.

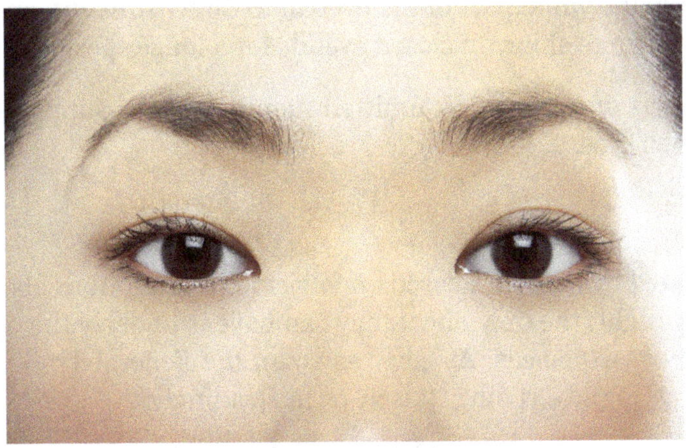

Eye movement exercises.

Perhaps finding Bates' concepts of "shifting" and "swinging" too complicated, some proponents of vision improvement, such as Bernarr Macfadden, suggested simply moving the eyes up and down, from side to side, and shifting one's gaze between a near-point and a far-point.

Sunning

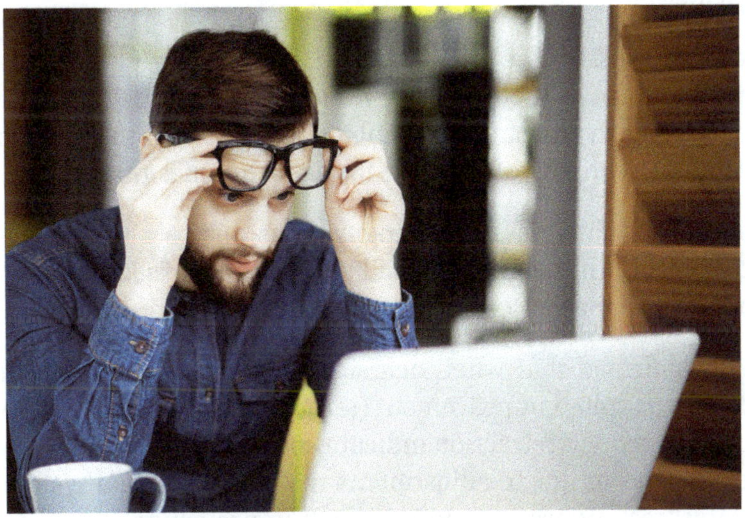

A burning-glass being used to focus sunlight on someone's eye, from Perfect Sight Without Glasses.

Bates believed that the eyes were benefited by exposure to sunlight. He stated that "persons with normal sight can look directly at the sun, or at the strongest artificial light, without injury or discomfort," and gave several examples of patients' vision purportedly improving after sungazing – this is at variance with the well-known risk of eye damage that can result from direct sunlight observation.

Bates said that, just as one should not attempt to run a marathon without training, one should not immediately look directly at the sun, but he suggested that it could be worked up to. He acknowledged that looking at the sun could have ill effects, but characterized them as being "always temporary" and in fact the effects of strain in response to sunlight. He wrote that he had cured people who believed that the sun had caused them permanent eye damage. In his magazine, Bates later suggested exposing only the white part of the eyeball to direct sunlight, and only for seconds at a time, after allowing the sun to shine on closed eyelids for a longer period.

Posthumous publications of Bates' book omitted mention of the supposed benefits from direct sunlight shining on open eyes.

Effectiveness

The techniques advocated by Bates are based on fallacious assumptions about the eye and have no effect on improving eyesight; the only effect they can have is to delay the use of effective therapy, with possible adverse consequences. As early as 1929, the Federal Trade Commission lodged a complaint against Bates' for advertising "falsely or misleadingly".

Philosopher Frank J. Leavitt has argued that the method Bates described would be difficult to test scientifically due to his emphasis on relaxation and visualization. Leavitt asked, "How can we tell whether someone has relaxed or imagined something, or just thinks that he or she has imagined it?" Regarding the possibility of a placebo trial, Leavitt commented, "I cannot conceive of how we could put someone in a situation where he thinks he has imagined something while we know that he has not."

Anecdotal Support

In support of the effectiveness of the Bates method, proponents point to the many accounts of people allegedly having improved their eyesight by applying it. While these anecdotes may be told and passed on in good faith, several potential explanations exist for the phenomena reported other than a genuine reversal of a refractive error due to the techniques practiced:

- Some cases of nearsightedness are recognized as due to a transient spasm of the ciliary muscle, rather than a misshapen eyeball. These are classed as pseudomyopia, of which spontaneous reversal may account for some reports of improvement.
- Research has confirmed that when nearsighted subjects remove their corrective lenses, over time there is a limited improvement (termed "blur adaptation") in their unaided visual resolution, even though refraction indicates no corresponding change in refractive error. This is believed to occur due to adjustments made in the visual system. One who has been practicing Bates' techniques and notices such improvement may not realize that simply leaving the glasses off would have had the same effect, which may be especially pronounced if the prescription was too strong to begin with.
- Visual acuity is affected by the size of the pupil. When it constricts (such as in response to an increase in light), the quality of focus will improve significantly, at the cost of a reduced ability to see in dim light. This is known as the "pinhole effect". This concept is also used in photography when changing the aperture size.
- Some eye defects may naturally change for the better with age or in cycles (ophthalmologist Stewart Duke-Elder suggested that this is what happened with Aldous Huxley). A cataract when first setting in sometimes results in much improved eyesight for a short time. One who happens to have been practicing the Bates method will likely credit it for any improvement experienced regardless of the actual cause.

- Some studies have suggested that a learned ability to interpret blurred images may account for perceived improvements in eyesight. Ophthalmologist Walter B. Lancaster had this to say: "Since seeing is only partly a matter of the image on the retina and the sensation it produces, but is in still larger part a matter of the cerebral processes of synthesis, in which memories play a principal role, it follows that by repetition, by practice, by exercises, one builds up a substratum of memories useful for the interpretation of sensations and facilitates the syntheses which are the major part of seeing." Lancaster faulted ophthalmologists in general for neglecting the role of the brain in the process of seeing, "leaving to irregular, half-trained workers the cultivation of that field".
- A 1952 study involving 100 subjects claiming to experience "flashes" of clear vision, in which eyesight momentarily becomes much sharper, found only one subject who "demonstrated unusually good transient acuity (a flash) but she was unable to maintain it or repeat it for measurement of refraction" and concluded that "'flashers' (those who can obtain remarkably large transient increases in visual acuity) are uncommon". A 2004 study proposed that such flashes may be caused by "negative accommodation" (i.e. an active flattening of the lens by the ciliary muscles).
- A 1982 study of subjects who underwent computer-based visual training concluded that any perceived resulting improvement in visual acuity is best explained as a contact lens-like effect of moisture on the eye, based on increased tear action exhibited by 15 out of 17 subjects who experienced such improvement.
- A 2003 study of claims that "positive suggestion (e.g., using hypnosis) can significantly improve visual acuity" found that "neither suggestion nor hypnotic phenomena are likely to significantly improve myopic vision".

Dead-end

A frequent criticism of the Bates method is that it has remained relatively obscure, which is seen as proof that it is not truly effective. Writer Alan M. MacRobert concluded in a 1979, that the "most telling argument against the Bates system" and other alternative therapies was that they "bore no fruit". In regards to the Bates method, he reasoned that "If palming, shifting, and swinging could really cure poor eyesight, glasses would be as obsolete by now as horse-drawn carriages."

Corrective Lenses and Safety

Discarding one's corrective lenses, as Bates recommended, or wearing lenses weaker than one's prescribed correction, as some Bates method advocates suggest, poses a potential safety hazard in certain situations, especially when one is operating a motor vehicle. James Randi related that his father, shortly after discarding glasses on the advice of Bates' book, wrecked his car. Bates method teachers often caution that when driving, one should wear the correction legally required.

Avoidance of Conventional Treatment

One of the greatest potential dangers of faith in the Bates method is that a believer may be disinclined to seek medical advice regarding what could be a sight-threatening condition requiring prompt treatment, such as glaucoma. Also, children with vision problems may require early attention by a professional in order to successfully prevent lazy eye. Such treatment may include exercises, but which are different from those associated with the Bates method, and parents who subscribe to Bates' ideas may delay seeking conventional care until it is too late. It may further be necessary for a child at risk of developing lazy eye to wear the proper correction.

ANIMAL-ASSISTED THERAPY

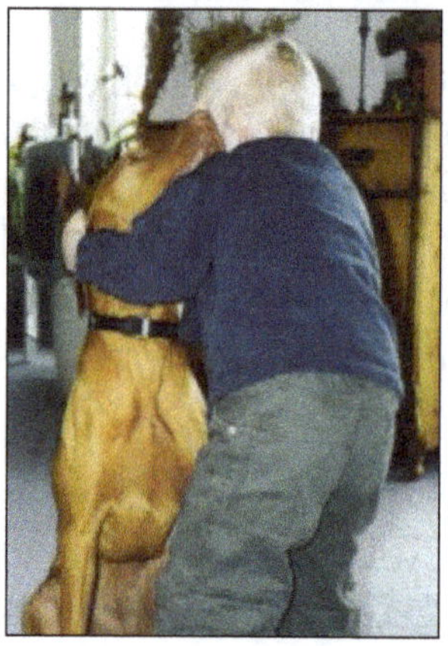

Dogs are common in animal-assisted therapy.

Animal-assisted therapy (AAT) is an alternative or complementary type of therapy that involves animals as a form of treatment. It falls under the realm of Animal Assisted Interventions (AAI). AAI is general term that encompasses any intervention or treatment that includes an animal in a therapeutic context such as Emotional-Support Animals, Service/Assistance Animals (i.e., trained animals that assist and support with daily activities), and Animal Assisted Activity (AAA). AAT contains sub-sections based on the type of animal, the targeted population, and how the animal is being incorporated into the therapeutic plan. The most commonly used types of AAT are canine-assisted therapy and equine-assisted therapy. The goal of AAT is to improve a patient's social, emotional, or cognitive functioning and literature reviews state that animals can be useful for educational and motivational effectiveness for participants. There are various studies documenting the positive effects of AAT reported through subjective self-rating scales and objective physiological measures, such as blood pressure, hormone levels, etc.

Physiological Effects

Wilson's (1984) biophilia hypothesis is based on the premise that our attachment to and interest in animals stems from the strong possibility that human survival was partly dependent on signals from animals in the environment indicating safety or threat. The biophilia hypothesis suggests that if we see animals at rest or in a peaceful state, this may signal to us safety, security and feelings of well-being which in turn may trigger a state where personal change and healing are possible.

Six neurotransmitters that influence mood have been documented to release after a 15-minute or more interaction with animals. Mirror neuron activity and disease-perception through olfactory (smelling) ability in dogs may also play important roles in helping dogs connect with humans during therapeutic encounters.

Medical Uses

Animals can be used in a variety of settings such as prisons, nursing homes, mental institutions, hospitals and in the home. Assistance dogs can assist people with many different disabilities; they are capable of assisting certain life activities and help the individuals navigate outside of the home.

As with all other interventions, assessing whether a program is effective as far as its outcomes are concerned is easier when the goals are clear and are able to be specified. There are a range of goals for animal assisted therapy programs relevant to children and young people, including enhanced capacity to form positive relationships with others. It is understood that pets provide benefits to those with mental health conditions, but further research is required to test the nature and extent of this relationship with an animal as a pet and how it differs between pets, emotional support animals, service animals, and animal-assisted therapy.

Cognitive Rehabilitation Treatment

Acquired Brain Injury (ABI) survivors with cognitive impairments can benefit from AAT as part of a comprehensive and holistic rehabilitation treatment plan.

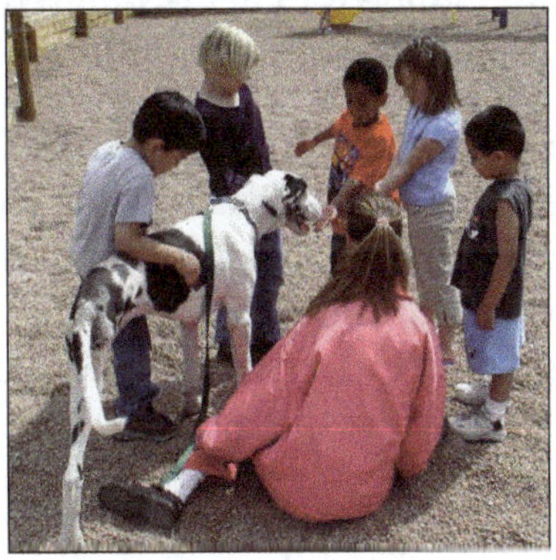

Pets may promote kindness in children.

Pediatric Care

Therapists rely on techniques such as monitoring a child's behavior with the animal, their tone of voice, and indirect interviewing. AAT can be used in children with mental health problems, can be used as a stand-alone treatment or it can be used along with conventional methods. Animals can be used as a distraction method when it comes to various situations or pain, and animals can also help bring happiness, pleasure, and entertainment to the pediatric population. Animals can also help improve children's moods and reinforce positive behaviors while helping to decrease negative ones. AAT research most commonly reported results were decreased anxiety and pain within the pediatric population. Dogs have shown to increase comfort and decrease pain in pediatric palliative care. Specific tactics have not been researched, but collective reviews of varied techniques displayed similar results of increased comfort reports by children and guardians.

Prisons

Animal-assistance programs may be useful in prisons to relieve stress of the inmates and workers, or to provide other benefits, but further study is needed to confirm the effectiveness of such programs in these settings. Internal file data reviews, anecdotal stories, and surveys of inmate and staff perceptions have been used to gauge the effectiveness of animal-assisted therapy in prisons, but these methods are limited and have resulted in an inadequate assessment.

Researchers have, however, begun to find methods of gauging the effectiveness of prison animal programs (PAP) by using Propensity Score Watching. Conclusions through this method showed that PAPs positively impact reductions in severe or violent infractions. A reduction in offenses statistically may reduce recidivism rates and increase former inmate job marketability and societal reintegration.

Inmates training and being responsible for an animal can foster empathy, emotional intelligence, communication, and self-control. PAP's also benefit the animals involved as many come from situations where they faced abuse, neglect or euthanasia.

Nursing Homes

The findings offer proof of the concept that canine-assisted therapies are feasible and can elicit positive quality-of-life experiences in institutionalized people with dementia. Researchers and practitioners need to elucidate the theoretical foundations of AATs. The Lived Environment Life Quality (LELQ) Model may serve as a guide for client-centered, occupation-focused, and ecologically valid approaches to animal-assisted occupational therapy beyond people with dementia.

When elderly people are transferred to nursing homes or LTC facilities, they often become passive, agitated, withdrawn, depressed, and inactive because of the lack of regular visitors or the loss of loved ones. Supporters of AAT say that animals can be helpful in motivating the patients to be active mentally and physically, keeping their minds sharp and bodies healthy. Therapists or visitors who bring animals into their sessions at the nursing home are often viewed as less threatening, which increases the relationship between the therapist/visitor and patient.

There are numerous techniques used in AAT, depending on the needs and condition of the patient. For elderly dementia patients, animal assisted therapy provides opportunities to have close physical contact with the animals, which may be helpful for people whose loved ones have passed and who do not frequently receive visitors.

Types

There are various animal species used in animal-assisted therapy (AAT). Individual animals are evaluated with strict criteria before being used in AAT. The criteria include appropriate size, age, aptitude, typical behaviors and the correct level of training. The most common forms of AAT are with dogs and horses. There is also published research on dolphin therapy.

Canine-assisted Therapy

In canine-assisted therapy, therapy dogs interact with clients in animal assisted interventions, to enhance therapeutic activities and well-being including the physical, cognitive, behavioral and socio-emotional functioning of clients. Well trained therapy dogs exhibit the behavior that human clients construe as friendly and welcoming. They comfort clients via body contact. Therapy dogs are also required to possess a calm temperament for accommodating the contact with unfamiliar clients while they serve as a source of comfort. They promote patients engaging in interactions which can help patient improve motor skills and establish trusting relationship with others. The interaction between patients and therapy dogs also aids reducing stressful and anxious feelings patients have. Due to those benefits, canine assisted therapy is used as a complement to other therapies to treat diagnosis such as post-traumatic stress disorder (PTSD), attention deficit hyperactivity disorder (ADHD), autism spectrum disorder (ASD), and dementia.

Canine assistance can also be used in classroom for promoting the development of creative writing and living skills and the participation of children in group activities. There are programs called canine-assisted reading programs which facilitate children with special educational needs. These programs utilize the calm, non-judgmental, happy characteristics of canines to let the process of reading become more meaningful and enjoyable for children. With these benefits, researchers suggest to incorporating dogs into assisting learning and educational programs.

Equine-related Therapy

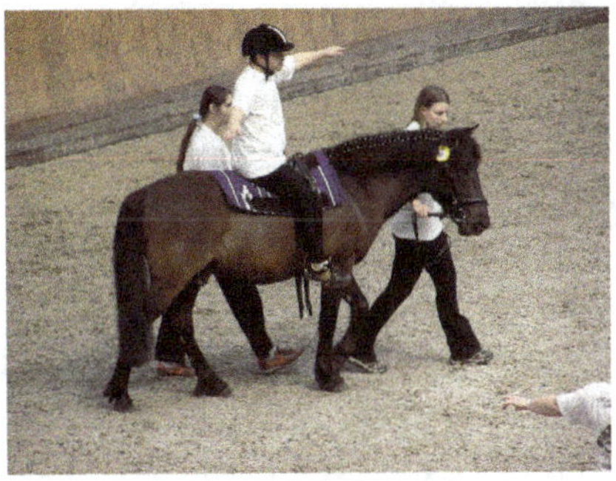

Hippotherapy is promoted as a treatment for people with physical or mental challenges.

A distinction exists between hippotherapy and therapeutic horseback riding. The American Hippotherapy Association defines hippotherapy as a physical, occupational, and speech-language therapy treatment strategy that utilizes equine movement as part of an integrated intervention program to achieve functional outcomes, while the Professional Association of Therapeutic Horsemanship International (PATHI) defines therapeutic riding as a riding lesson specially adapted for people with special needs. According to Marty Becker, hippotherapy programs are active "in twenty-four countries and the horse's functions have expanded to therapeutic riding for people with physical, psychological, cognitive, social, and behavioral problems". Hippotherapy has also been approved by the American Speech and Hearing Association as a treatment method for individuals with speech disorders. In addition, equine assisted psychotherapy (EAP) uses horses for work with persons who have mental health issues. EAP often does not involve riding.

Dolphin Therapy

Dolphin assisted therapy refers to the controversial alternative medicine practice of swimming with dolphins. This form of therapy has been strongly criticized as having no long term benefit, and being based on flawed observations. Psychologists have cautioned that dolphin assisted therapy is not effective for any known condition and presents considerable risks to both human patients and the captive dolphins. The child has a one-on-one session with a therapist in a marine park of some kind. An ethical issue with data on dolphin-assisted therapy and the effectiveness of it is that most of the research is done by people who operate the dolphin-assisted therapy programs.

Conditions Benefit from Animal-assisted Therapy

Based on current research, there are many conditions/disorders that can benefit from animal-assisted therapy (AAT) in diverse settings around the world. Those conditions include psychological disorder, developmental disorder, dementia, cancer, chronic pain, advanced heart failure, etc. Animal-assisted therapy is commonly used for psychological disorder. Disorders such as attention deficit hyperactivity disorder(ADHD), autism spectrum disorder(ASD), post-traumatic stress disorder(PTSD), major depressive disorder (MDD) are part of psychological disorders that can benefit from animal-assisted therapy.

Effectiveness

In recent decades, an increased number of research indicates the social, psychological, and physiological benefits of animal assisted therapy in health and education field. Although the effectiveness of AAT is still unclear due to the lack of clarity regarding the degree to which the canine itself contributes in the recovery process, there is a growing awareness that AAT may be effective in treating attention deficit hyperactivity disorder, post-traumatic stress disorder, autism spectrum disorder, and dementia.

Attention Deficit Hyperactivity Disorder

Children with attention deficit hyperactivity disorder (ADHD) may decrease behavioral issues and improve socialization skills with the intervention of AAT. Compared to children only received cognitive-behavioral therapy (CBT), children who received both canine-assisted therapy and cognitive-behavioral therapy (CBT) had reduce in severity of ADHD symptoms. However, the canine-assisted therapy had no effect on relieving ADHD symptoms in long-term treatment.

Post-traumatic Stress Disorder

Animal-assisted Therapy for the Treatment of Trauma in Military Veterans

Post-traumatic stress disorder (PTSD) is a psychological disorder affects people's mental health and has varying severity and forms. PTSD is often difficult to treat due to high drop-out rates and low responses to traditional psychotherapeutic approaches and interventions.

Animals have two types of effects, direct and indirect, on a mental health spectrum including biological, psychological, and social responses, further targeting marked symptoms of PTSD (i.e., re-experiencing, avoidance, changes in beliefs/feelings, and hyperarousal). Direct effects of animals include a decrease in anxiety and blood pressure while indirect effects result in increased social interactions and overall participation in everyday activities.

Biologically, specific neurochemicals are released when observing human and animal interactions. Similarly, dog assistance can potentially mediate oxytocin which effects social and physical well-being and decrease blood pressure. The psychological benefits of animals focus mainly on dog and human interactions, the reduction of anxiety and depressive symptoms, and increased resilience. Animals in this capacity can further provide emotional and psychological assistance and support, addressing several PTSD symptoms. The presence of an animal can alleviate intrusion symptoms by providing a reminder that there is no danger present. Animals can further elicit positive emotions, targeting emotional numbing experiences. Animal interactions also provide social benefits, providing companionship and alleviate feelings of loneliness and isolation through everyday routines and increased social interactions in public.

The incorporation and involvement of animals dates back to the earliest forms of organized combat. Dogs, in particular, were utilized in different capacities. Ancient armies employed dogs as Soldiers and companions which extended to modern combat including dogs as a crucial asset in communication, detection, and intimidation. In World War II, dogs were used in therapy as emotional support during the war. While a range of animals can be utilized in AAIs, dogs and horses have been investigated and explored as forms of rehabilitation for veterans suffering from PTSD. Dog assisted therapy and therapeutic horseback riding are non-invasive methods for treating post-traumatic stress disorder (PTSD) in veterans..

Canines can easily integrate into a multitude of environments, are highly responsive to humans, and are very intelligent. For those reasons, dogs are the most common animal used in AAIs. Dogs are typically categorized according to the level of training received and the specific needs of the individual. A service dog provides relief through specialized support related to a physical, mental, or psychological disability. Emotional support animals (ESAs) solely provide psychological relief and do not require specialized training. Therapy animals often provide additional support in a therapeutic environment by supporting counselors or therapists in their therapeutic duties. While service dogs, ESAs, and therapy dogs can support the diverse symptoms that veterans, specifically bred and selected dogs, PTSD Service Dogs (PSDs), are trained and assigned to veterans with PTSD to support with daily life activities as well as with emotional and mental health needs.

Dogs provide subjective positive effects to veterans and serve as a compassionate reminder to veterans suffering from PTSD that danger is not present, creating a safe space for the veteran. They are often sensitive to humans and have the ability to adapt their behavior accordingly by doing tasks such as preventing panic, waking a veteran from a nightmare, and nudging to help the veteran "stay in the present". Dogs also provide veterans with a nonjudgmental and safe environment that can help a veteran express feelings and process thoughts without interruption, criticism or advice. Interactions, such as petting, playing and walking, with the dog can increase physical activity, reduce anxiety, and provide encouragement to stay in the present moment. The interaction between dog and veterans supports social interactions for isolated veterans, reduces symptoms associated with PTSD such as depression and anxiety, and increases veterans' calmness.

Similar to dogs, horses have been included in the treatment of veterans suffering from PTSD by providing an accepting and nonjudgmental environment, which further facilitates a veterans' ability to cope with symptoms associated with PTSD. Because horses are social animals, they are capable of creating and responding to relationships based on the veteran's energy, providing an opportunity for veterans to regain the ability to form trusting relationships. Therapeutic work with horses varies from ground-based activities, mounted activities, or a combination of both. In the therapeutic context, horses can promote cognitive reframing as well as an increase in the use of mindfulness practice. While there is limited research and standardized instruments to measure the effects, veterans who have participated in pilot programs have better communicate skills, self-awareness, and self-esteem, promoting safety and support during the transition into civilian life. Long term effects of equine based interventions with veterans include increased happiness, social support, and better sleep hygiene because they are able to process information regarding their emotions and behaviors in a nonjudgmental space.

While AAIs can be effective, they also have limitations due to limited research and findings on AAIs and veterans with PTSD.Furthermore, studies approved yield small sample sizes which limit the power to detect changes as well as the specific tasks that are particularly helpful to veterans. AAT may alsoobstruct veterans from cultivating their own way of control over stressful situation.

Autism Spectrum Disorder

AAT could reduce the symptoms of ASD such as aggressiveness, irritability, distractibility, and hyperactivity. In one review, five out of nine studies reviewed showed positive effects of therapeutic horseback riding on children with ASD. Canine assisted intervention provides a calmer environment by reducing the stress, irritation, and anxiety that children with ASD experience. Playing with dogs increases the positive mood in children with ASD. Animals also can serve as a social catalyst. In the presence of animals, children with ASD are more likely engage in social interactions with humans. However, the impact of AAT upon parent-child interaction is not clear.

Dementia

AAT encourages expressions of emotions and cognitive stimulation through discussions and reminiscing of memories while the patient bonds with the animal. A study in 2017 evaluated results from ten researches and found that animal assisted therapies (particularly using dogs) resulted in measurable quality of life improvements for patients with dementia. Patients with dementia were also found to improve their social interactions and their scores on the Cohen-Mansfield Agitation Inventory (CMAI).

Limitations

There is limited scientific research on the use of AAT within the population of adults who have been sexually assaulted. While animals do tend to comfort victims, animal therapy may not be the catalyst that provides positive success in therapy sessions. As mentioned above, adults tend not to focus as much on having an animal companion, and therefore, animal therapy cannot be attributed as the reason for success in those types of therapy sessions. There are some ethical concerns that arise when applying animal therapy to younger victims of sexual assault. For example, if a child is introduced to an animal that is not their pet, the application of animal therapy can cause some concerns. First of all, some children may not be comfortable with animals or may be frightened which could be avoided by asking permission to use animals in therapy. Second, a special bond is created between animal and child during animal therapy. Therefore, if the animal in question does not belong to the child, there may be some negative side effects when the child discontinues therapy. The child will have become attached to the animal, which does raise some ethical issues as far as subjecting a child to the disappointment and possible relapse that can occur after therapy discontinues.

Another limitation of animal assisted therapy is that AAT might be a short term reinforce, not a long term one.

The effectiveness of AAT is also still unclear due to the lack of clarity regarding the degree to which the canine itself contributes in the recovery process.

There are some concerns specific to dolphin-assisted therapy: First, it is potentially hazardous to the human patients, and it is harmful to the dolphins themselves; by taking dolphins out of their natural environment and putting them in captivity for therapy can be hazardous to their well-being. Second, dolphin-assisted therapy has been strongly criticized as having no long term benefit, and being based on flawed observations. Third, psychologists have cautioned that dolphin assisted therapy is not effective for any known condition.

DETOXIFICATION

Detoxification is a type of alternative-medicine treatment which aims to rid the body of unspecified "toxins" – substances that proponents claim have accumulated in the body and have undesirable short-term or long-term effects on individual health. Activities commonly associated with detoxification include dieting, fasting, consuming exclusively or avoiding specific foods (such as fats, carbohydrates, fruits, vegetables, juices, herbs, or water), colon cleansing, chelation therapy, and the removal of dental fillings containing amalgam.

Scientists and health organizations have criticized the concept of detoxification for its unsound scientific basis and for the lack of evidence for claims made. The "toxins" usually remain undefined, with little to no evidence of toxic accumulation in the patient. The British organisation Sense About Science has described some detox diets and commercial products as "a waste of time and money", while the British Dietetic Association called the idea "nonsense" and a "marketing myth". Dara Mohammadi summarizes "detoxing" as "a scam a pseudo-medical concept designed to sell you things".

Suspicions of the inefficacy of purging became widespread by the 1830s. Biochemistry and microbiology appeared to support auto-intoxication theory in the 19th century, but by the early twentieth century detoxification-based approaches quickly fell out of favour. Even though abandoned by mainstream medicine, the idea has persisted in the popular imagination and amongst alternative medicine practitioners. Notions of internal cleansing had resurgence along with the rise of alternative medicine in the 1970s and following; it remains unscientific and anachronistic. With the rise of the environmentalist movement, many detox diets use the diet format as a political platform to advocate for environmental ideas about pollution and toxic contamination.

Types

Detox Diets

Detox diets are dietary plans that claim to have detoxifying effects. The general idea suggests that most food contains contaminants: ingredients deemed unnecessary for human life, such as flavor enhancers, food colorings, pesticides, and preservatives. Scientists, dietitians, and doctors, while generally viewing "detox diets" as harmless (unless nutritional deficiency results), often dispute the value and need of "detox diets", due to lack of supporting factual evidence or coherent rationale. In cases where a person suffers from a disease, belief in the efficacy of a detox diet can result in delay or failure to seek effective treatment.

Detox diets can involve consuming extremely limited sets of foods (only water or juice, for example, a form of fasting known as juice fasting), eliminating certain foods (such as fats) from the diet, or eliminating processed foods and alleged irritants. Detox diets are often high in fiber. Proponents claim that this causes the body to burn accumulated stored fats, releasing fat-stored "toxins" into the blood, which can then be eliminated through the blood, skin, urine, feces and breath. Proponents claim that things such as an altered body-odor support the notion that detox diets have an effect. The mainstream medical view is that the body has mechanisms to rid itself of toxins, and a healthy diet is best for the body. Although a brief fast of a single day is unlikely to cause harm, prolonged fasting (as recommended by certain detox diets) can have dangerous health consequences or can even be fatal.

Colon Cleansing

Colon cleansing involves giving an enema (colonic) containing some salt, and sometimes coffee or herbs to remove food that, according to proponents, remains in the colon, producing nonspecific symptoms and general ill-health. However, the colon usually does not require any help cleaning itself. The practice can be potentially dangerous if incorrectly practised.

Heavy Metals

Practitioners may recommend detoxification as a treatment to address the notion that mercury poisoning arises from consumption of contaminated fish and from dental amalgam fillings – Quackwatch states: "Removing good fillings is not merely a waste of money. In some cases, it results in tooth loss because when fillings are drilled out, some of the surrounding tooth structure will be removed with it."

Detoxification Devices

Certain devices are promoted to allegedly remove toxins from the body. One version involves a foot-bath using a mild electric current, while another involves small adhesive pads applied to the skin (usually the foot). In both cases, the production of an alleged brown "toxin" appears after a brief delay. In the case of the foot bath, the "toxin" is actually small amounts of rusted iron leaching from the electrodes. The adhesive pads change color due to oxidation of the pads' ingredients in response to the skin's moisture. In both cases, the same color-changes occur irrespective of whether the water or patch even make contact with the skin (they merely require water—thus proving the color-change does not result from any body-detoxification process).

Colon Cleansing

Colon cleansing (also known as colon therapy) encompasses a number of alternative medical therapies claimed to remove nonspecific toxins from the colon and intestinal tract by removing any accumulations of feces. Colon cleansing may be branded colon hydrotherapy, a colonic or colonic irrigation. During the 2000s Internet marketing and infomercials of oral supplements supposedly for colon cleansing increased. Colon cleansing in this context should not be confused with an enema which introduces fluid into the colon under mainstream medical supervision for a limited number of purposes including severe constipation or medical imaging.

Some forms of colon hydrotherapy use tubes to inject water, sometimes mixed with herbs or with other liquids, into the colon via the rectum using special equipment. Oral cleaning regimens use dietary fiber, herbs, dietary supplements, or laxatives. People who practice colon cleansing believe that accumulations of putrefied feces line the walls of the large intestine and that these accumulations harbor parasites or pathogenic gut flora, causing nonspecific symptoms and general ill-health. This "auto-intoxication" hypothesis is based on medical beliefs of the Ancient Egyptians and was discredited in the early 20th century.

There is no scientific evidence for the alleged benefits of colon cleansing. Certain enema preparations have been associated with heart attacks and electrolyte imbalances, and improperly prepared or used equipment can cause infection or damage to the bowel. Frequent colon cleansing can lead to dependence on enemas to defecate and some herbs may reduce the effectiveness of, or increase the risks associated with the use of prescription medications.

Effectiveness and Risks

The symptoms that are attributed to auto-intoxication headache, fatigue, loss of appetite and irritability may be caused by mechanical distention within the bowel, such as irritable bowel syndrome, rather than toxins from putrefying food. The benefits anecdotally attributed to colon cleansing are vague and the claims made by manufacturers and practitioners are based on a flawed understanding of the body. There is little evidence of actual benefit to the procedure, and no evidence that it can alleviate the symptoms that are attributed to the theories of colon cleansing.

As the colon normally expels waste, colon cleansing is generally unneeded. Colonic irrigation can disrupt the bowel's normal flora, and, if done frequently, can result in electrolyte depletion with dehydration. Rare but severe adverse events have been rectal perforation, as well as amoebic infection, from poorly sterilised equipment. Others claim that colon cleansing may impede the colon's shedding of dead cells.

Excessive use of enemas has also been associated with heart problems, such as heart failure, as well as heart attacks related to electrolyte imbalances when performed as a coffee enema. Frequent enemas or other colon-cleansing tools may lead to dependence and inability to defecate without assistance, as well as potential withdrawal symptoms. Herbs taken orally may modulate the absorption or the activity of prescription medications.

Medical doctor Harriet Hall writes that "The colon cleanses itself". The idea that its walls are coated with years-old hamburger residue is preposterous".

Colon Hydrotherapy

Colonic irrigation also known as colon hydrotherapy, colonic hydrotherapy, or a "colonic", is a treatment which is used "to wash out the contents of the large bowel by means of copious enemas using water or other medication."

During an enema, the water is retained in the colon for approximately 15 minutes. During a colonic, water is introduced into the colon and then it is flushed out and this is repeated until the entire colon is cleared.

Colonic irrigation has been described as an "unwise" procedure as it carries the risk of serious harm and has no proven benefit.

Supplement Effectiveness

The consumer advocacy news program marketplace conducted a consumer trial with three women on the effectiveness of two colon supplements versus fiber. The results showed the supplements did not assist in weight loss and provided no additional benefit over a basic fiber supplement. According to the American Cancer Society, "Available scientific evidence does not support claims that colon therapy is effective in treating cancer or any other disease".

ALTERNATIVE CANCER TREATMENTS

Alternative cancer treatments are alternative or complementary treatments for cancer that have not been approved by the government agencies responsible for the regulation of therapeutic goods. They include diet and exercise, chemicals, herbs, devices, and manual procedures. The treatments are not supported by evidence, either because no proper testing has been conducted, or because testing did not demonstrate statistically significant efficacy. Concerns have been raised about the safety of some of them. Some treatments that have been proposed in the past have been found in clinical trials to be useless or unsafe. Some of these obsolete or disproven treatments continue to be promoted, sold, and used. Promoting or marketing such treatments is illegal in most of the developed world including the United States and European Union.

A distinction is typically made between complementary treatments which do not disrupt conventional medical treatment, and alternative treatments which may replace conventional treatment. Alternative cancer treatments are typically contrasted with experimental cancer treatments – which are treatments for which experimental testing is underway – and with complementary treatments, which are non-invasive practices used alongside other treatment. All approved chemotherapeutic cancer treatments were considered experimental cancer treatments before their safety and efficacy testing was completed.

Since the 1940s, medical science has developed chemotherapy, radiation therapy, adjuvant therapy and the newer targeted therapies, as well as refined surgical techniques for removing cancer. Before the development of these modern, evidence-based treatments, 90% of cancer patients died within five years. With modern mainstream treatments, only 34% of cancer patients die within five years. However, while mainstream forms of cancer treatment generally prolong life or permanently cure cancer, most treatments also have side effects ranging from unpleasant to fatal, such as pain, blood clots, fatigue, and infection. These side effects and the lack of a guarantee that treatment will be successful create appeal for alternative treatments for cancer, which purport to cause fewer side effects or to increase survival rates despite evidence to suggest a 2.5 fold increase in death with alternative medicines.

Alternative cancer treatments have not undergone properly conducted, well-designed clinical trials. Among those that have been published, the methodology is often poor.

Prevalence

Survey data about how many cancer patients use alternative or complementary therapies vary from nation to nation as well as from region to region. A 2000 study evaluated a sample of 1023 women from a British cancer registry suffering from breast cancer and found that 22.4% had consulted with a practitioner of complementary therapies in the previous twelve months. The study concluded that the patients had spent many thousands of pounds on such measures and that use "of practitioners of complementary therapies following diagnosis is a significant and possibly growing phenomenon".

In Australia, one study reported that 46% of children suffering from cancer have been treated with at least one non-traditional therapy. Further 40% of those of any age receiving palliative care had tried at least one such therapy. Some of the most popular alternative cancer treatments were found to be dietary therapies, antioxidants, high dose vitamins, and herbal therapies.

Use of unconventional cancer treatments in the United States has been influenced by the U.S. federal government's National Center for Complementary and Alternative Medicine (NCCAM), initially known as the Office of Alternative Medicine (OAM), which was established in 1992 as a National Institutes of Health (NIH) adjunct by the U.S. Congress. More specifically, the NIC's Office of Cancer Complementary and Alternative Medicine sponsors over $105 million a year in grants for pseudoscientific cancer research. Over thirty American medical schools have offered general courses in alternative medicine, including the Georgetown, Columbia, and Harvard university systems, among others.

People who Choose Alternative Treatments

People who choose alternative treatments tend to believe that evidence-based medicine is extremely invasive or ineffective, while still believing that their own health could be improved. They are loyal to their alternative healthcare providers and believe that "treatment should concentrate on the whole person".

Cancer patients who choose alternative treatments instead of conventional treatments believe themselves less likely to die than patients who choose only conventional treatments. They feel a greater sense of control over their destinies, and report less anxiety and depression. They are more likely to engage in benefit finding, which is the psychological process of adapting to a traumatic situation and deciding that the trauma was valuable, usually because of perceived personal and spiritual growth during the crisis.

However, patients who use alternative treatments have a poorer survival time, even after controlling for type and stage of disease. In 2017, researchers at Yale School of Medicine published a paper which suggested that people who choose alternative medicine over conventional cancer treatments were more than twice as likely to die within five years of diagnosis. And specifically, in those with breast cancer, people choosing alternative medicine were 5.68 times more likely to die within five years.

The reason that patients using alternative treatments die sooner may be because patients who accurately perceive that they are likely to survive do not attempt unproven remedies, and patients who accurately perceive that they are unlikely to survive are attracted to unproven remedies. Among patients who believe their condition to be untreatable by evidence-based medicine, "desperation drives them into the hands of anyone with a promise and a smile." Con artists have long exploited patients' perceived lack of options to extract payments for ineffectual and even harmful treatments.

In a survey of American cancer patients, baby boomers were more likely to support complementary and alternative treatments than people from an older generation. White, female, college-educated patients who had been diagnosed more than a year ago were more likely than others to report a favorable impression of at least some complementary and alternative benefits.

Questionable and Ineffective Treatments

Many therapies have been (and continue to be) promoted to treat or prevent cancer in humans but lack good scientific and medical evidence of effectiveness. In many cases, there is good scientific evidence that the alleged treatments do not work. Unlike accepted cancer treatments, unproven and disproven treatments are generally ignored or avoided by the medical community, and are pseudoscientific.

Despite this, many of these therapies have continued to be promoted as effective, particularly by promoters of alternative medicine. Scientists consider this practice quackery, and some of those engaged in it have been investigated and prosecuted by public health regulators such as the US Federal Trade Commission, the Mexican Secretariat of Health and the Canadian Competition Bureau. In the United Kingdom, the Cancer Act makes the unauthorized promotion of cancer treatments a criminal offense.

Specific Methods

- Curcumin.
- Deoxycholic acid.
- Dichloroacetic acid.
- HuaChanSu, traditional Chinese medicine extracted from the skin of the Bufo toad.
- Medical cannabis (especially for “Appetite Stimulation” and “Analgesia”).
- Melittin (via “Nanobees”).
- Milk thistle.
- Proton therapy.
- Selenium (Selenomethionine and *Se*-methylselenocysteine).

Pain Relief

Most studies of complementary and alternative medicine in the treatment of cancer pain are of low quality in terms of scientific evidence. Studies of massage therapy have produced mixed results, but overall show some temporary benefit for reducing pain, anxiety, and depression and a very low risk of harm, unless the patient is at risk for bleeding disorders. There is weak evidence for a modest benefit from hypnosis, supportive psychotherapy and cognitive therapy. Results about Reiki and touch therapy were inconclusive. The most studied such treatment, acupuncture, has demonstrated no benefit as an adjunct analgesic in cancer pain. The evidence for music therapy is equivocal, and some herbal interventions such as PC-SPES, mistletoe, and saw palmetto are known to be toxic to some cancer patients. The most promising evidence, though still weak, is for mind–body interventions such as biofeedback and relaxation techniques.

Examples of Complementary Therapy

As stated in the scientific literature, the measures listed below are defined as 'complementary' because they are applied in conjunction with mainstream anti-cancer measures such as chemotherapy, in contrast to the ineffective therapies viewed as 'alternative' since they are offered as substitutes for mainstream measures.

- Acupuncture may help with nausea but does not treat the disease.
- Psychotherapy may reduce anxiety and improve quality of life as well as allow for improving patient moods.
- Massage therapy may temporarily reduce pain.
- There is no evidence that cannabis has a beneficial effect in preventing or treating cancer in humans.
- Hypnosis and meditation may improve the quality of life of cancer patients.
- Music therapy eases cancer-related symptoms by helping with mood disturbances.

Alternative Theories of Cancer

Some alternative cancer treatments are based on unproven or disproven theories of how cancer begins or is sustained in the body. Some common concepts are:

- Mind-body connection: This idea says that cancer forms because of, or can be controlled through, the person's mental and emotional state. Treatments based on this idea are mind–body interventions. Proponents say that cancer forms because the person is unhappy or stressed, or that a positive attitude can cure cancer after it has formed. A typical claim is that stress, anger, fear, or sadness depresses the immune system, whereas that love, forgiveness, confidence, and happiness cause the immune system to improve, and that this improved immune system will destroy the cancer. This belief that generally boosting the immune system's activity will kill the cancer cells is not supported by any scientific research. In fact, many cancers require the support of an active immune system (especially through inflammation) to establish the tumor microenvironment necessary for a tumor to grow.
- Toxin theory of cancer: In this idea, the body's metabolic processes are overwhelmed by normal, everyday byproducts. These byproducts, called "toxins", are said to build up in the cells and cause cancer and other diseases through a process sometimes called autointoxication or autotoxemia. Treatments following this approach are usually aimed at detoxification or body cleansing, such as enemas.
- Low activity by the immune system: This claim asserts that if only the body's immune system were strong enough, it would kill the "invading" or "foreign" cancer. Unfortunately, most cancer cells retain normal cell characteristics, making them appear to the immune

system to be a normal part of the body. Cancerous tumors also actively induce immune tolerance, which prevents the immune system from attacking them.

- Epigenetic disregulation. This claim uses research into the mechanism of epigenetics to understand how mutations in the epigenetic machinery of cells will altered histone acetylation patterns to create cancer epigenetics. DNA damage appears to be the primary underlying cause of cancer. If DNA repair is deficient, DNA damage tends to accumulate. Such excess DNA damage can increase mutational errors during DNA replication due to error-prone translesion synthesis. Excess DNA damage can also increase epigenetic alterations due to errors during DNA repair. Such mutations and epigenetic alterations can give rise to cancer.

HYDROTHERAPY

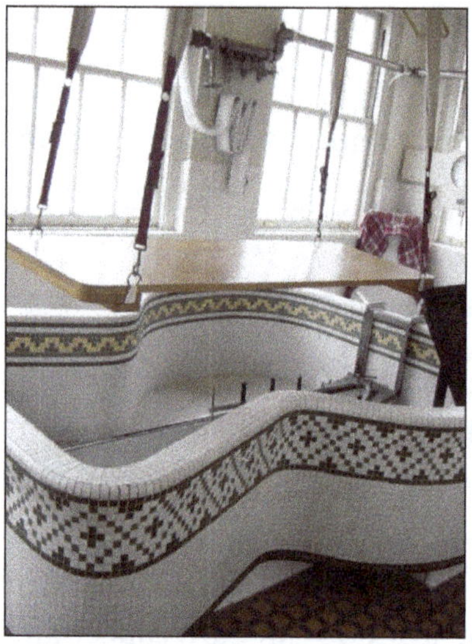

Hubbard Tub with wooden patient lift.

Hydrotherapy, formerly called hydropathy and also called water cure, is a part of alternative medicine (particularly naturopathy), occupational therapy, and physiotherapy, that involves the use of water for pain relief and treatment. The term encompasses a broad range of approaches and therapeutic methods that take advantage of the physical properties of water, such as temperature and pressure, for therapeutic purposes, to stimulate blood circulation and treat the symptoms of certain diseases.

Various therapies used in the present day hydrotherapy employ water jets, underwater massage and mineral baths (e.g. balneotherapy, Iodine-Grine therapy, Kneipp treatments, Scotch hose, Swiss shower, thalassotherapy) or whirlpool bath, hot Roman bath, hot tub, Jacuzzi, cold plunge and mineral bath.

The therapeutic use of water has been recorded in ancient Egyptian and Roman civilizations. Egyptian royalty bathed with essential oils and flowers, while Romans had communal public baths for their citizens. Hippocrates prescribed bathing in spring water for sickness. Other cultures noted for a long history of hydrotherapy include China and Japan, the latter being centred primarily around Japanese hot springs or "onsen". Many such histories predate the Roman thermae.

Modern Revival

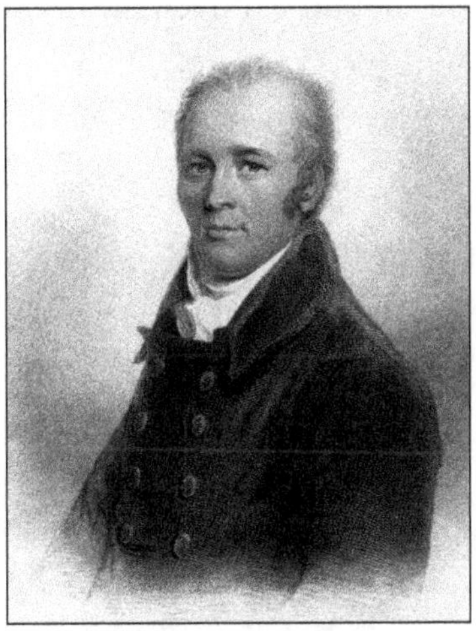

James Currie.

An important note on the growth of hydropathy is that it started to become prominent as traditional medical practice was becoming more professional in terms of how doctors operated, alienating many patients, as they felt that the medical encounter was becoming less personalized, and the more scientific the medical language became, the less that they could easily understand. Hydropathy was a return to a treatment that was spiritual and natural, making it more palatable to those who felt uncomfortable with the direction that traditional medicine was taking.

The general idea behind hydropathy during the 1800s was to be able to induce something called a crisis. The thinking was that water invaded any cracks, wounds, or imperfections in the skin, which were filled with impure fluids. Health was considered to be the natural state of the body, and filling these spaces with pure water, would flush the impurities out, which would rise to the surface of the skin, producing pus. The event of this pus emerging was called a crisis, and was achieved through a multitude of methods. These methods included techniques such as sweating, the plunging bath, the half bath, the head bath, the sitting bath, and the douche bath. All of these were ways to gently expose the patient to cold water in different ways.

Two English works on the medical uses of water were published in the 18th century that inaugurated the new fashion for hydrotherapy. One of these was by Sir John Floyer, a physician of Lichfield, who, struck by the remedial use of certain springs by the neighbouring peasantry, investigated the history of cold bathing and published a book on the subject in 1702. The book ran through six editions within a few years and the translation of this book into German was largely drawn upon by Dr J. S. Hahn of Silesia as the basis for his book called On the Healing Virtues of Cold Water, Inwardly and Outwardly Applied, as Proved by Experience, published in 1738.

The other work was a 1797 publication by Dr James Currie of Liverpool on the use of hot and cold water in the treatment of fever and other illness, with a fourth edition published in 1805, not long before his death. It was also translated into German by Michaelis (1801) and Hegewisch (1807). It was highly popular and first placed the subject on a scientific basis. Hahn's writings had meanwhile created much enthusiasm among his countrymen, socictics having been formed everywhere to promote the medicinal and dietetic use of water; and in 1804 Professor E.F.C. Oertel of Anspach republished them and quickened the popular movement by unqualified commendation of water drinking as a remedy for all diseases.

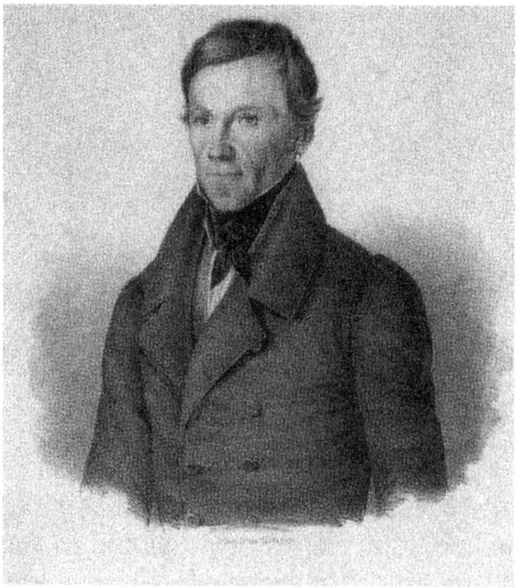

Vincenz Priessnitz.

Vincent Preissnitz

Vincent Preissnitz was the son of a peasant farmer who, as a young child, observed a wounded deer bathing a wound in a pond near his home. Over the course of several days, he would see this deer return and eventually the wound was healed. Later as a teenager, Preissnitz was attending to a horse cart, when the cart ran him over, breaking three of his ribs. A physician told him that they would never heal. Preissnitz decided to try his own hand at healing himself, and wrapped his wounds with damp bandages. By daily changing his bandages and drinking large quantities of water, after about a year, his broken ribs had been cured. Preissnitz quickly gained fame in his hometown and became the consulted physician.

Later in life, Preissnitz became the head of a hydropathy clinic in Gräfenberg in 1826. He was extremely successful and by 1840, he had 1600 patients in his clinic including many fellow physicians, as well as important political figures such as nobles and prominent military officials. Treatment length at Preissnitz's clinic varied. Much of his theory was about inducing the above mentioned crisis, which could happen quickly, or could occur after three to four years. In accordance with the simplistic nature of hydropathy, a large part of the treatment was based on living a simple lifestyle. These lifestyle adjustments included dietary changes such as eating only very coarse food, such as jerky and bread, and of course drinking large quantities of water. Preissnitz's treatments also included a great deal of less strenuous exercise, mostly including walking. Ultimately, Preissnitz's clinic was extremely successful, and he gained fame across the western world. His practice even influenced the hydropathy that took root overseas in America.

Sebastian Kneipp

Sebastian Kneipp was born in Germany and he considered his own role in hydropathy to be that of continuing Preissnitz's work. Kneipp's own practice of hydropathy was even gentler than the norm. He believed that typical hydropathic practices deployed were "too violent or too frequent" and he expressed concern that such techniques would cause emotional or physical trauma to the patient. Kneipp's practice was more all encompassing than Preissnitz's, and his practice involved not only curing the patients' physical woes, but emotional and mental as well.

Kneipp introduced four additional principles to the therapy: medicinal herbs, massages, balanced nutrition, and "regulative therapy to seek inner balance". Kneipp had a very simple view of an already simple practice. For him, hydropathy's primary goals were strengthening the constitution and removing poisons and toxins in the body. These basic interpretations of how hydropathy worked hinted at his complete lack of medical training. Kneipp did have, however, a very successful medical practice in spite of, perhaps even because of, his lack of medical training. As mentioned above, some patients were beginning to feel uncomfortable with traditional doctors because of the elitism of the medical profession. The new terms and techniques that doctors were using were difficult for the average person to understand. Having no formal training, all of his instructions and published works are described in easy to understand language and would have seemed very appealing to a patient who was displeased with the direction traditional medicine was taking.

A significant factor in the popular revival of hydrotherapy was that it could be practised relatively cheaply at home. The growth of hydrotherapy (or 'hydropathy' to use the name of the time), was thus partly derived from two interacting spheres: "the hydro and the home".

Hydrotherapy as a formal medical tool dates from about 1829 when Vincenz Priessnitz, a farmer of Gräfenberg in Silesia, then part of the Austrian Empire, began his public career in the paternal homestead, extended so as to accommodate the increasing numbers attracted by the fame of his cures.

At Gräfenberg, to which the fame of Priessnitz drew people of every rank and many countries, medical men were conspicuous by their numbers, some being attracted by curiosity, others by the desire of knowledge, but the majority by the hope of cure for ailments which had as yet proved incurable. Many records of experiences at Gräfenberg were published, all more or less favorable to the claims of Priessnitz, and some enthusiastic in their estimate of his genius and penetration.

Spread of Hydrotherapy

Captain R. T. Claridge was responsible for introducing and promoting hydropathy in Britain, first in London in 1842, then with lecture tours in Ireland and Scotland in 1843. His 10-week tour in Ireland included Limerick, Cork, Wexford, Dublin and Belfast, over June, July and August 1843, with two subsequent lectures in Glasgow.

Some other Englishmen preceded Claridge to Graefenberg, although not many. One of these was Dr. James Wilson, who himself, along with Dr James Manby Gully, established and operated a water cure establishment at Malvern in 1842. In 1843, Wilson and Gully published a comparison of the efficacy of the water-cure with drug treatments, including accounts of some cases treated at

Malvern, combined with a prospectus of their Water Cure Establishment. Then in 1846 Gully published The Water Cure in Chronic Disease, further describing the treatments available at the clinic.

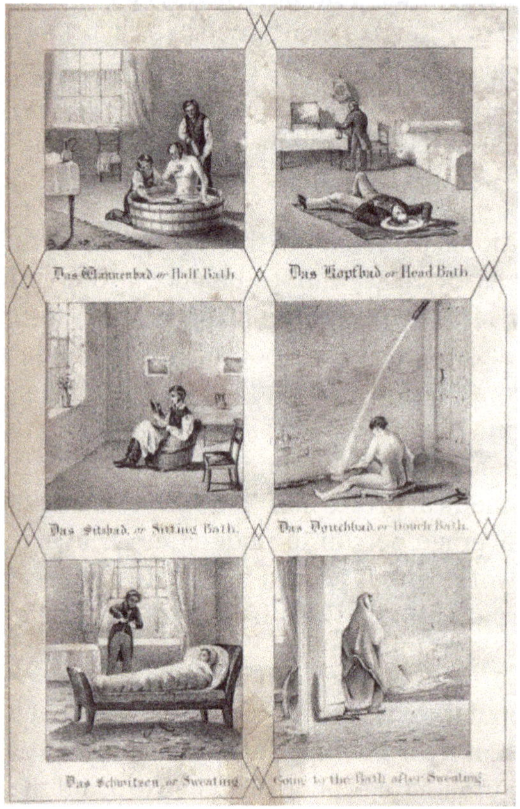

Hydropathic applications according to Claridge's Hydropathy book.

The fame of the water-cure establishment grew, and Gully and Wilson became well-known national figures. Two more clinics were opened at Malvern. Famous patients included Charles Darwin, Charles Dickens, Thomas Carlyle, Florence Nightingale, Lord Tennyson and Samuel Wilberforce. With his fame he also attracted criticism: Sir Charles Hastings, a physician and founder of the British Medical Association, was a forthright critic of hydropathy, and Gully in particular.

From the 1840s, hydropathics were established across Britain. Initially, many of these were small institutions, catering to at most dozens of patients. By the later nineteenth century the typical hydropathic establishment had evolved into a more substantial undertaking, with thousands of patients treated annually for weeks at a time in a large purpose-built building with lavish facilities – baths, recreation rooms and the like – under the supervision of fully trained and qualified medical practitioners and staff.

In Germany, France and America, and in Malvern, England, hydropathic establishments multiplied with great rapidity. Antagonism ran high between the old practice and the new. Unsparing condemnation was heaped by each on the other; and a legal prosecution, leading to a royal commission of inquiry, served but to make Priessnitz and his system stand higher in public estimation.

Increasing popularity soon diminished caution whether the new method would help minor ailments and be of benefit to the more seriously injured. Hydropathists occupied themselves mainly with studying chronic invalids well able to bear a rigorous regimen and the severities of unrestricted crisis. The need of a radical adaptation to the former class was first adequately recognized by John Smedley, a manufacturer of Derbyshire, who, impressed in his own person with the severities as well as the benefits of the cold water cure, practised among his workpeople a milder form of hydropathy, and began about 1852 a new era in its history, founding at Matlock a counterpart of the establishment at Gräfenberg.

Ernst Brand of Berlin, Raljen and Theodor von Jürgensen of Kiel, and Karl Liebermeister of Basel, between 1860 and 1870, employed the cooling bath in abdominal typhus with striking results, and led to its introduction to England by Dr Wilson Fox. In the Franco-German War the cooling bath was largely employed, in conjunction frequently with quinine; and it was used in the treatment of hyperpyrexia.

Hot Baths

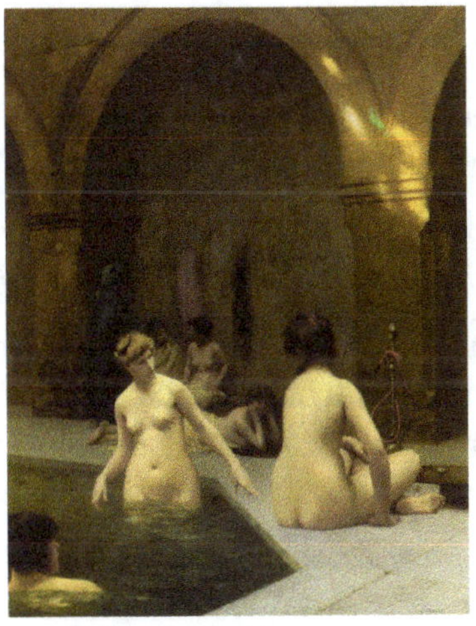

Baigneuses, oil on canvas.

Hydrotherapy, especially as promoted during the height of its Victorian revival, has often been associated with the use of cold water, as evidenced by many titles from that era. However, not all therapists limited their practice of hydrotherapy to cold water, even during the height of this popular revival.

The specific use of heat was however often associated with the Turkish bath. This was introduced by David Urquhart into England on his return from the East in the 1850s, and ardently adopted by Richard Barter. The Turkish bath became a public institution, and, with the morning tub and the general practice of water drinking, is the most noteworthy of the many contributions by hydropathy to public health.

Spread to the United States

The first U.S. hydropathic facilities were established by Joel Shew and Russell Thacher Trall in the 1840s. Dr Charles Munde also established early hydrotherapy facilities in the 1850s.

By 1850, it was said that "there are probably more than one hundred" facilities, along with numerous books and periodicals, which had "attained an extent of circulation equalled by few monthlies in the world". By 1855, there were attempts by some to weigh the evidence of treatments in vogue at that time.

Following the introduction of hydrotherapy to the U.S., John Harvey Kellogg employed it at Battle Creek Sanitarium, which opened in 1866, where he strove to improve the scientific foundation for hydrotherapy. Other notable hydropathic centers of the era included the Cleveland Water Cure Establishment, founded in 1848, which operated successfully for two decades, before being sold to an organization which transformed it into an orphanage.

At its height, there were over 200 water-cure establishments in the United States, most located in the northeast. Few of these lasted into the postbellum years, although some survived into the 20th century including institutions in Scott (Cortland County), Elmira, Clifton Springs and Dansville. While none were located in Jefferson County, the Oswego Water Cure operated in the city of Oswego.

Subsequent Developments

Hydropathy was a specific instance, or "particular case", of general principles of thermodynamics. That is, "the application of heat and cold in general", as it applies to physiology, mediated by hydropathy. In 1883, another writer stated "Not, be it observed, that hydropathy is a water treatment after all, but that water is the medium for the application of heat and cold to the body".

Hydrotherapy was used to treat people with mental illness in the 19th and 20th centuries and before World War II, various forms of hydrotherapy were used to treat alcoholism. The basic text of the Alcoholics Anonymous fellowship, Alcoholics Anonymous, reports that A.A. co-founder Bill Wilson was treated by hydrotherapy for his alcoholism in the early 1930s.

Recent Techniques

A subset of cryotherapy involves cold water immersion or ice baths, used by physical therapists, sports medicine facilities and rehab clinics. Proponents assert that it results in improved return of blood flow and byproducts of cellular breakdown to the lymphatic system and more efficient recycling.

Alternating the temperatures, either in a shower or complementary tanks, combines the use of hot and cold in the same session. Proponents claim improvement in circulatory system and lymphatic drainage. Experimental evidence suggests that contrast hydrotherapy helps to reduce injury in the acute stages by stimulating blood flow and reducing swelling

Uses

Water therapy may be restricted to use as aquatic therapy, a form of physical therapy, and as a cleansing agent. However, it is also used as a medium for delivery of heat and cold to the body, which has long been the basis for its application. Hydrotherapy involves a range of methods and techniques, many of which use water as a medium to facilitate thermoregulatory reactions for therapeutic benefit.

Hydrotherapy is used as an adjunct to therapy, including in nursing, where its use is now long established. It continues to be widely used for burn treatment, although shower-based hydrotherapy techniques have been increasingly used in preference to full-immersion methods, partly for the ease of cleaning the equipment and reducing infections due to contamination. When removal of tissue is necessary for the treatment of wounds, hydrotherapy which performs selective mechanical debridement can be used. Examples of this include directed wound irrigation and therapeutic irrigation with suction.

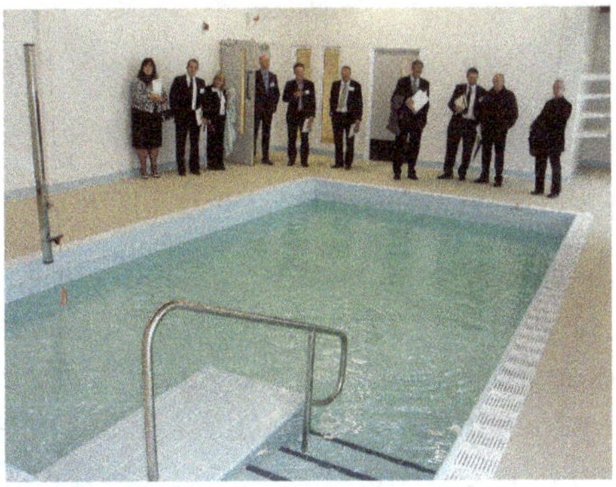

Opening of the new Hydrotherapy Pool.

Technique

The appliances and arrangements by means of which heat and cold are brought to bear are (a) packings, hot and cold, general and local, sweating and cooling; (b) hot air and steam baths; (c) general baths, of hot water and cold; (d) sitz (sitting), spinal, head and foot baths; (e) bandages (or compresses), wet and dry; also (f) fomentations and poultices, hot and cold, sinapisms, stupes, rubbings and water potations, hot and cold.

Hydrotherapy which involves submerging all or part of the body in water can involve several types of equipment:

- Full body immersion tanks (a "Hubbard tank" is a large size).
- Arm, hip, and leg whirlpool.

Whirling water movement, provided by mechanical pumps, has been used in water tanks since at least the 1940s. Similar technologies have been marketed for recreational use under the terms "hot tub" or "spa".

In some cases baths with whirlpool water flow aren't used to manage wounds because a whirlpool will not selectively target the tissue to be removed and can damage all tissue. Whirlpools also create an unwanted risk of bacterial infection, can damage fragile body tissue, and in the case of treating arms and legs, bring risk of complications from edema.

OZONE THERAPY

Ozone therapy is a form of alternative medicine that purports to increase the amount of oxygen in the body through the introduction of ozone. Various techniques have been suggested, with purported benefits including the treatment of cancer, AIDS, and multiple sclerosis, among others.

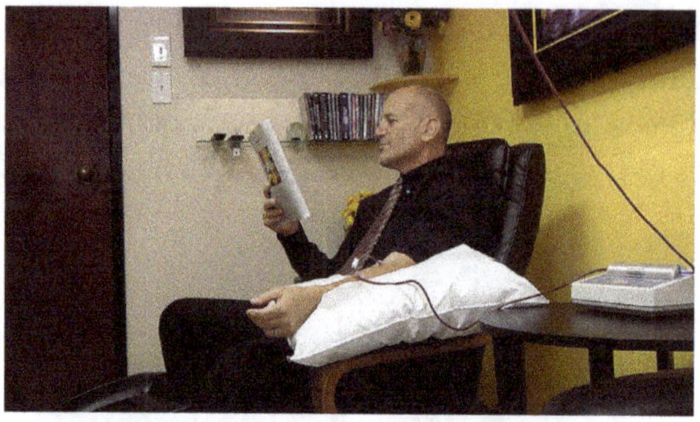

Person undergoing ozone IV therapy.

Ozone therapy is sold as an alternative treatment for various illnesses. Beginning in 1991 the FDA has prosecuted and sent to jail several people presenting themselves as medical doctors and selling ozone therapy products as a medical cure or operating medical clinics using ozone therapy for healing human illness. Arrests following similar activity have been made in other countries as well. At least 10 deaths have been related to ozone therapy or its lack of usefulness, in nine cases there had been investigation and in eight it was discovered that the practitioners had used false credentials.

In 1856, just 16 years after its discovery, ozone was first used in a health care setting to disinfect operating rooms and sterilize surgical instruments. By the end of the 19th century the use of ozone to disinfect drinking water of bacteria and viruses was well established in mainland Europe.

The administration of ozone for treatment of tuberculosis. During World War I, ozone was tested at Queen Alexandra Military Hospital in London as a possible disinfectant for wounds. The gas was applied directly to wounds for as long as 15 minutes. This resulted in damage to both bacterial cells and human tissue. Other sanitizing techniques, such as irrigation with antiseptics, were found preferable.

In April 2016, the FDA prohibited the medical use of ozone, "In any medical condition for which there is no proof of safety and effectiveness", stating "Ozone is a toxic gas with no known useful medical application in specific, adjunctive, or preventive therapy. In order for ozone to be effective as a germicide, it must be present in a concentration far greater than that which can be safely tolerated by man and animals."

Proposed Uses

Ozone therapy consists of the introduction of ozone into the body via various methods, usually involving its mixture with various gases and liquids before injection, with potential routes including the vagina, rectum, intramuscular (in a muscle), subcutaneously (under the skin), or intravenously (directly into veins). Ozone can also be introduced via autohemotherapy, in which blood is drawn from the patient, exposed to ozone and re-injected into the patient.

Ozone therapy as a safe and low-cost method, could provide promising results among women with mild to moderate CTS, at least for short-term treatment.

This therapy has been proposed for use in various diseases, including cancer, AIDS, multiple sclerosis, arthritis, heart disease, Alzheimer's dementia, and Lyme disease, though supportive evidence for these applications is limited. Theories about the ability of ozone to kill tumor cells with oxygen have no credible scientific basis. For treatment of HIV/AIDS, although ozone deactivates the viral particles outside the body, there is no evidence of benefit for living patients.

The United States Food and Drug Administration initially stated in 1976, and reiterated its position in 2006, that when inhaled, ozone is a toxic gas which has no demonstrated safe medical application, though their position statements primarily deal with its potential for causing inflammation and pulmonary edema in the lungs. They also emphasize that in order for ozone to be effective as a germicide, it must be present at concentrations far greater than can be safely tolerated by humans or other animals. More recent reviews have highlighted that different routes of administration may result in different therapeutic and side effect profiles, though a statistically robust meta analysis of available research has not been performed to date.

Ozone has been suggested for use in dentistry, but existing evidence does not support its use.

Some reviews have suggested ozone as potential treatment for herniated discs and diabetic neuropathy.

There is some controversy about its use by athletes in an attempt to increase performance; although its use is not disallowed in and of itself, it can be mixed with banned substances for administration prior to injection.

Safety

Much of the concern related to ozone therapy revolves around the safety of blood ozonation. It is well established that when inhaled by mammals, ozone reacts with compounds in tissues lining the lungs and triggers a cascade of pathological effects including pulmonary edema. Saul Green has argued that since ozone has the capacity to oxidize organic compounds in an atmospheric environment, it should also logically oxidize blood components and endogenous human tissues. High levels of inhaled ozone are known to be toxic, though single-dose inhalation of lower levels is not. Proponents suggest that its effects are tissue dependent, though the subject is still debated.

Serious complications reported from the use of this therapy include the development of hepatitis and also include five reported fatalities. There is some concern about an association with heart attacks after autohemotherapy, though this association has been contested as well.

NEURAL THERAPY

Neural therapy is a form of alternative medicine in which local anesthetic is injected into certain locations of the body in an attempt to treat chronic pain and illness.

There is no good evidence that the therapy works and it carries some risk; it has not been found to be of overall benefit.

Neural therapy has been described as a form of holistic medicine for treating illness and chronic pain. According to Quackwatch, neural therapy is "a bizarre approach claimed to treat pain and disease by injecting local anesthetics into nerves, scars, glands, trigger points, and other tissues".

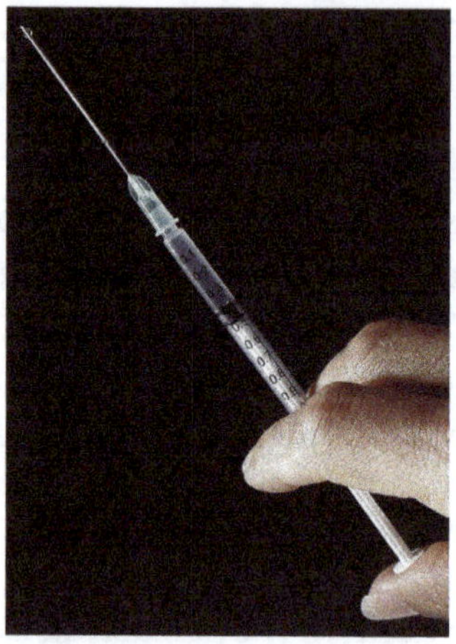

In neural therapy anaesthetic is injected to try and disrupt a type of electrical energy said to cause illness.

The idea underlying the therapy is that "interference fields" (*Störfelder*) at certain sites of the body are responsible for a type of electric energy that causes illness. The fields can be disrupted by injection, allowing the body to heal.

The practice originated in 1925 when Ferdinand Huneke, a German surgeon, used a newly launched pain drug that contained procaine (a local anaesthetic) on his sister who had severe intractable migraines. Instead of using it intramuscularly as recommended he injected it intravenously and the migraine attack stopped immediately. He and his brother Walter subsequently used Novocaine in a similar way to treat a variety of ailments.

In 1940 Ferdinand Huneke injected the painful shoulder of a woman who also had an osteomyelitis in her leg which at that time (before antibiotics) threatened her with amputation. The shoulder pain improved somewhat but the leg wound became itchy. On injecting the leg wound the shoulder pain vanished immediately – a reaction he called the "phenomenon of seconds" (Sekundenphänomen).

Reception, Effectiveness and Safety

Neural therapy is practiced mostly in South America and Europe. A 2007 survey of family physicians in Germany found neural therapy to be among the most used of alternative medical techniques.

Quackwatch includes neural therapy on its list of "questionable treatments".

According to the American Cancer Society, "available scientific evidence does not support claims that neural therapy is effective in treating cancer or any other disease". Overall the risks of the treatment, such as of needle damage to organs, outweigh any benefit it may have.

CHIROPRACTIC

Chiropractic is a system of diagnosis and treatment based on the concept that the nervous system coordinates all of the body's functions, and that disease results from a lack of normal nerve function.

Chiropractic employs manipulation and adjustment of body structures, such as the spinal column, so that pressure on nerves coming from the spinal cord due to displacement (subluxation) of a vertebral body may be relieved. Practitioners believe that misalignment and nerve pressure can cause problems not only in the local area, but also at some distance from it. Chiropractic treatment appears to be effective for muscle spasms of the back and neck, tension headaches, and some sorts of leg pain. It may or may not be useful for other ailments.

Modern chiropractic was founded by Daniel David Palmer, a grocer, who performed his first chiropractic adjustment in 1895.

Not all chiropractors are alike in their practice. The International Chiropractors Association believes that patients should be treated by spinal manipulation alone while the American Chiropractors Association advocate a multidisciplinary approach that combines spinal adjustment with other modalities such as physical therapy, psychological counseling, and dietary measures.

Chiropractic Adjustment

A chiropractic back adjustment is a type of manual therapy (i.e., a treatment delivered through the physician's hands) that seeks to realign joint subluxations. Note that the word subluxation means different things to a chiropractor than it does to a medical doctor, though either way, the definition of the term is "partial dislocation."

When a chiropractor looks for a subluxation (via the diagnostic process,) the things she notes tend to be subtle gradations of position changes in the joints and accompanying soft tissue problems. When a medical doctor sees a subluxation on an x-ray, it's a very obvious disconnect between the bones that make up a joint.

Learn more about the difference between the way an allopathic doctor sees a subluxation vs the way a chiropractor sees it.

Although a number of chiropractic methods and techniques exist, the most common version of an adjustment involves a controlled but fast directional thrust into the joint.

The goal is to bring the bones of a joint back to their normal, natural fit. It may take just one adjustment to achieve this aim (so that the adjustment "sticks,") or it may take several.

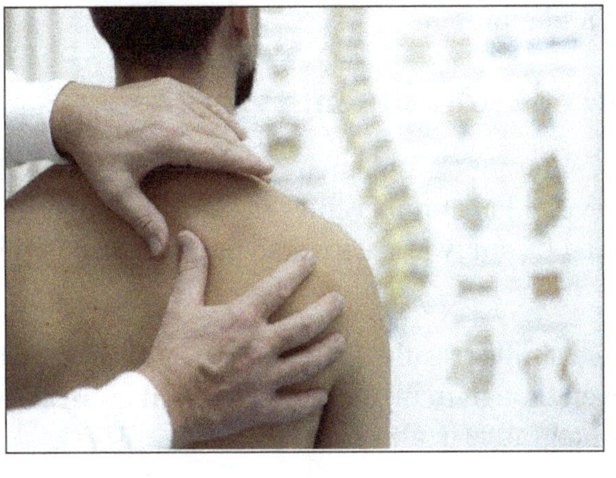

Other more industry related names for a chiropractic adjustment are: spinal manipulation and Grade 5 mobilization. Physical therapists and osteopathic physicians are two other types of health providers who are sometimes trained and licensed to give a Grade 5 mobilization treatment.

Grades 1-4 type mobilizations are less forceful and direct than Grade 5 and tend to be used more by physical therapists, massage therapists and some holistic therapists and educators such as Feldenkrais practitioners, Alexander teachers and more. Massage therapists, athletic trainers, personal trainers and holistic practitioners are, in general, not licensed to give spinal manipulation therapy, i.e., Grade 5 mobilization.

A Reputation for Back Cracking

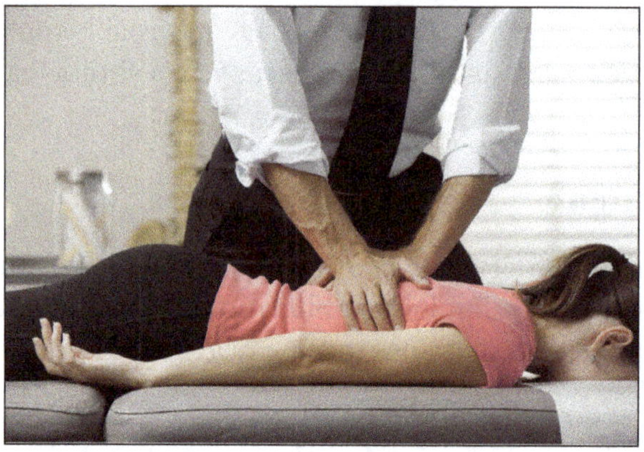

You probably already know that chiropractors are often referred to as "back crackers." This nickname may have been bestowed based on the cracking and popping that's usually heard during a treatment.

A lot of people associate these sounds with a successful adjustment. But in reality, they may have nothing to do with accurate re-alignment of your joints. Instead, they are thought to be a result of cavitation, which is a sudden pressure decrease inside the joint (brought about by the manipulation.) Cavitation causes gasses in the synovial fluid to be released into the space between the bones that are being adjusted (called the joint space.)

And while it's true that the mainstay of the chiropractic profession is adjustment of the spine, most also adjust the pelvis as a routine part of the treatment. Some also regularly adjust other joints such as knees, feet, wrists, and more.

How Well do Chiropractic Adjustments Work?

According to the National Center for Complementary and Integrative Health (NCCIH), spinal manipulation is one among several holistic therapies that has been proven to provide low back pain relief. Pain relief experienced by study participants who underwent chiropractic adjustments was mild and moderate.

Other holistic therapies yield similar results include massage therapy and exercise. Physical therapy is on this list, as well, even though many people think of it as an allied health profession, rather than a complementary or integrative health field.

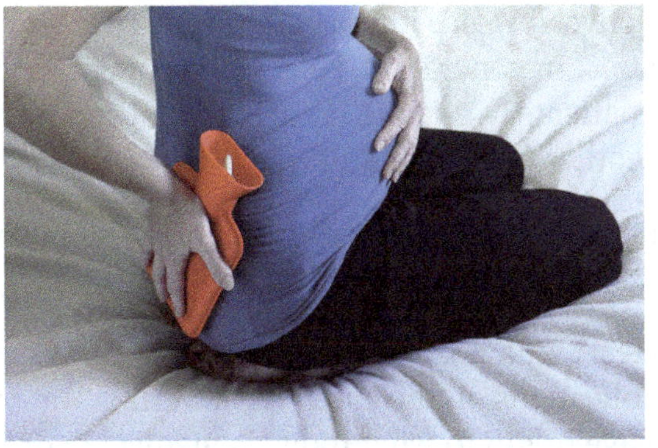

If you have chronic low back pain, and you want to get it treated by a chiropractor (or osteopath or physical therapist who performs spinal manipulation,) A review found high quality evidence that this treatment is just as good as other treatments for the same condition. Such comparison treatments included the use of heat, sleeping on a firm mattress and/or taking pain relievers.

BALNEOTHERAPY

The balneotherapy is effective for the treatment of many diseases. It can relieve your symptoms if you suffer osteoarthritis, fibromyalgia, Rheumatoid arthritis, among other conditions of the musculoskeletal system. Therefore, it is usually used in physiotherapy.

It can also be useful in the treatment of various skin conditions, including psoriasis, acne and dermatitis.

Characteristics of Balneotherapy

Within what is considered balneotherapy are various treatments or therapies involving baths with sea water, river water, hot springs or waters with a high content of mineral salts.

In addition to the immersion baths, massage with water in motion and relaxation or stimulation exercises performed with water or water, are also considered part of balneotherapy.

In spas, complex buildings specially designed to offer these treatments, there are usually steam baths, common saunas and dry saunas, as part of balneotherapy. In some cases the treatment may include the intake of these waters.

Treatments with medicinal clays, rich in mineral salts, are often combined with balneotherapy and can be considered part of this discipline. These sludges are usually obtained from rivers, lakes or lagoons.

One of the advantages of clay therapy is that take a long time to cool, so that it is easier to combine mineral therapy with thermal therapy.

It is important to emphasize that all these treatments must be supervised by properly trained personnel. Ideally, when entering a Spa, be a doctor who evaluates your personal situation, your general health, and then indicate the best treatment for you.

For balneotherapy to be effective, it is also important to lead a healthy life, with a balanced diet and sports and recreation activities. In general the spas are located in regions with a pleasant natural environment, which allows patients to contact nature, so that can be more relaxed and in this way make the most of your balneotherapy treatments.

Balneotherapy is nothing new, there are indications that it was already used by the ancient Romans and other peoples.

Since the time of Hippocrates Y Galen the power and importance of healing waters and baths is known. In 1473, the first publications on the cures with thermal water, which were true treaties of balneotherapy, and which gave origin to what today is medical hydrology, that is, the application of different waters as treatment for certain diseases.

In the nineteenth century balneotherapy had its greatest boom, due to the lack of drugs for many diseases. Almost all conditions that had no specific treatment, were treated with thermal water and many medical researchers at that time recorded a large number of techniques and Applications of balneotherapy.

In Italy, for example, the use of hot springs for curative purposes has ancient origins, but even today there is a number of spas that apply hot springs from the bowels of the earth (especially in volcanic areas) for the treatment of various conditions.

Medicinal Mineral Waters

In most cases, the waters used in balneotherapy treatments contain a certain concentration of mineral salts. Depending on what these salts are, the therapeutic effects of these waters may be different.

For example, in sulphated water, the sulfate anion is the predominant one. This type of water favors bowel movements and liver functioning, therefore, are frequently used in the treatment of diseases of the digestive system.

In the chlorinated water, on the other hand, the chloride anion predominates, although there may also be a similar concentration of sodium. These Waters are applied in patients with respiratory disorders and skin conditions, as they have an anti-inflammatory and disinfectant effect.

The sulphurous waters, with high content of hydrogen sulfide, have an anti-allergic and antirheumatic effect. They are used for treatment of rheumatic and dermatological conditions.

Waters with high calcium salts have anti-inflammatory, anti-allergic and sedative properties.

The waters with presence of baking soda can be administered orally and are useful in the treatment of heartburn, gastritis and hernia hiatus among others, due to its antacid effect.

On the other hand, waters with carbon dioxide, naturally or added by man can stimulate the secretion of juices gastricos that favor the digestion, if they are ingested as part of a balneotherapy treatment.

Waters with a certain concentration of iron may have a positive effect on patients with fragile nails and hair, due to their regenerative properties.

He water with radon, which is a source of weak radioactive emissions, can be drunk, inhaled or used in baths for the treatment of degenerative or inflammatory diseases of the joints and vascular diseases.

In order for water from a spring to be considered useful for balneotherapy treatments it must have a salt concentration equal to or greater than 1 gram per liter. Most of these types of waters arise with a certain temperature, although not all the waters applied in balneotherapy are hot springs.

Techniques Applied in Balneotherapy

The most frequent are the balneotherapy treatments in which the water is applied topically, for example, in immersion baths .

For example, if you go to a spa you may be placed in a bath filled with water at a temperature between 34 and 37 degrees, for about 15 to 20 minutes. Then you'll have a break of about half an hour, covered with sheets or blankets so you do not cool down suddenly.

Another common technique is the application of water springs under pressure, as in a whirlpool. With this type of treatment, in addition to benefits of water rich in minerals, also the positive effects of the mechanical action of the jets are obtained.

These techniques stimulate the blood circulation, help increase vascularization and promote muscle relaxation, which can achieve a some analgesia (relief of pain) and improves the mobility of the locomotor system.

Other treatments include wraps, underwater massages, irrigations, among others.

Some waters with a high mineral content can to drink Always under medical indication, although it is not the most frequent treatment. With this therapy it is possible to stimulate kidney function, improve digestion and intestinal mobility.

Finally, these mineral waters can also enter the body through inhalation, in a sauna for example, or even by mcans of Inhalers or nebulizers.

What do the Scientific Studies Say?

Balneotherapy is traditionally known for providing relief to joint pain, relaxing muscles, favoring oxygenation of tissues, decrease stress and for its use in beauty treatments.

There are several scientific studies that have shown the positive effects of balneotherapy in patients with different conditions. Although the researchers believe that further studies are needed, the positive results that have already been achieved are very encouraging.

Balneotherapy in Patients with Rheumatoid Arthritis

Another review of studies on the effect of balneotherapy in patients with rheumatoid arthritis, the results of which were published in 2015, concluded that"the positive findings in most studies can not be ignored,"but they also point out that research in this regard.

Studies suggest that balneotherapy treatments can decrease pain and improve joint mobility in this type of patients.

Balneotherapy in Patients with Osteoarthritis

In 2008, the results of many investigations on the effects of balneotherapy in patients with osteoarthritis were reviewed and found

- High-mineral water immersion baths can alleviate pain and improve the quality of life of patients (by comparison with a control group that received no treatment).
- The baths in sulfur waters and baths of immersion with dead sea water are also able to relieve the pain after a month of treatment, also compared to another group of patients who did not receive any treatment.

The great advantage of balneotherapy treatments is that, in most cases, they do not have adverse side effects, unlike virtually all medications usually prescribed for pain relief in this type of patients.

Balneotherapy for Psoriasis and Atopic Dermatitis

In the area of dermatology, balneotherapy also has important applications. Positive effects have been seen in patients with psoriasis and atopic dermatitis .

Although the mechanism by which water with minerals has a curative effect on the skin is not known, it is believed that this could be due to a combination of chemical, thermal, mechanical and immunoregulatory effects.

Again, one of the main advantages of balneotherapy is that it does not imply any type of medicine that is potentially toxic or harmful side effects.

If you submit to a balneotherapy treatment, there are practically no risks to your health and well-being, and you may get very positive effects if atopic dermatitis or psoriasis.

Scientists recommend using balneotherapy as a complementary treatment to medications or as Only treatment if with the medicines you have not managed to improve much.

Baths with Dead Sea Water in Patients with Fibromyalgia

The effects of balneotherapy in patients with fibromyalgia have been well studied by the scientific community through various investigations, all with very positive results.

In one of these investigations, 48 patients were treated with fibromyalgia and underwent balneotherapy with dead sea water (water sulphurated), in a spa on the shores of the mentioned sea. The therapy lasted 10 days.

The overall condition of the patients was evaluated before starting treatment, after ten days of therapy, one month after the end of treatment and three months later.

In patients receiving treatment, a significant improvement in fibromyalgia symptoms was observed. The patients had less fatigue, lower levels of anxiety, less headaches, sleep problems and joint pains. And best of all is that these positive effects are remained after three months of therapy.

Another scientific study revealed that balneotherapy is also capable of improving respiratory function in this type of patients. in a study carried out of 56 people, who received complementary therapy with balneotherapy, had significant improvements in their symptoms. Dyspnoea and in their spirometry, even six months after the end of treatment, which lasted three weeks.

That is why scientists recommend balneotherapy (if it can be with dead sea water, better) as a complementary treatment in patients with fibromyalgia, that disease whose symptoms are so difficult to alleviate.

As you can see, balneotherapy is an effective treatment in many diseases, and its effects have been scientifically proven.

If you are suffering from joint pains due to osteoarthritis, rheumatoid arthritis or fibromyalgia, balneotherapy may be an excellent option for you. The even if you have psoriasis or atopic dermatitis and you have not been able to relieve yourself with conventional treatment.

HALOTHERAPY

Halotherapy is an alternative treatment that involves breathing salty air. Some claim that it can treat respiratory conditions, such as asthma, chronic bronchitis, and allergies. Others suggest it can also:

- Ease smoking-related symptoms, such as a cough, shortness of breath, and wheezing.
- Treat depression and anxiety.
- Cure some skin conditions, such as psoriasis, eczema, and acne.

The origins of halotherapy date back to the medieval era. But researchers only recently started studying its potential benefits.

Halotherapy Methods

Halotherapy is usually broken down into dry and wet methods, depending on how the salt is administered.

Dry Methods

The dry method of halotherapy is usually done in a man-made "salt cave" that's free of humidity. The temperature is cool, set to 68 °F (20 °C) or lower. Sessions usually last for about 30 to 45 minutes.

A device called a halogenerator grinds salt into microscopic particles and releases them into the air of the room. Once inhaled, these salt particles are claimed to absorb irritants, including allergens and toxins, from the respiratory system. Advocates say this process breaks up mucus and reduces inflammation, resulting in clear airways.

The salt particles are said to have a similar effect on your skin by absorbing bacteria and other impurities responsible for many skin conditions.

Salt is also said to produce negative ions. This theoretically causes your body to release more serotonin, one of the chemicals behind feelings of happiness. Many people use Himalayan salt lamps to get the benefits of negative ions at home. However, there's no evidence that these lamps have any benefit other than adding ambience.

Wet Methods

Halotherapy is also done using a mixture of salt and water. Wet methods of halotherapy include:

- Gargling salt water.
- Drinking salt water.
- Bathing in salt water.
- Using salt water for nasal irrigation.
- Flotation tanks filled with salt water.

Does Halotherapy have any Risks?

Halotherapy is probably safe for most people, but there aren't any studies on its safety. In addition, halotherapy is usually done in a spa or wellness clinic without trained medical staff on hand to handle medical emergencies. Keep this in mind as you weigh the pros and cons of halotherapy.

While it's said to treat asthma, halotherapy might also constrict or irritate the airwaves in people with asthma. This can make coughing, wheezing, and shortness of breath worse. Some people also report getting headaches during halotherapy.

Halotherapy is a complementary therapy that's meant to work with any medications you're on. Let your doctor know you want to try this approach. Don't stop any medications without discussing it with your doctor.

Supporters of halotherapy claim it's safe for children and pregnant women. However, there's little research to back up this claim. According to a 2008 study, inhaling a 3 percent saline solution is a safe and effective treatment for infants with bronchiolitis. However, there's no standardization across halotherapy clinics. The amount of salt administered can vary greatly.

Halotherapy may be a relaxing spa treatment, but there's little evidence about how well it works. Some research suggests that it may be beneficial for respiratory problems and depression.

References

- The-benefits-of-acupressure: verywellhealth.com, Retrieved 21 May, 2019
- Gorski, david. "battlefield acupuncture revisited: that's it? That's all col. Niemtzow's got?". Science-based medicine. Retrieved 19 july 2014
- Dugan, dan (2002-01-01). Michael shermer (ed.). Anthroposophy and anthroposophical medicine. The skeptic encyclopedia of pseudoscience. Abc-clio. Pp. 31–32. Isbn 978-1-57607-653-8
- Acupuncture-in-cardiology, acupuncture-in-modern-medicine: intechopen.com, Retrieved 5 February, 2019
- Lee ms, shin bc, suen lk, park ty, ernst e (2008). "auricular acupuncture for insomnia: a systematic review". Int. J. Clin. Pract. (systematic review). 62 (11): 1744–52. Doi:10.1111/j.1742-1241.2008.01876.x. Pmid 18754807

- Offit, paul a. (2011). Deadly choices: how the anti-vaccine movement threatens us all. Basic books. P. 13. Isbn 978-0-465-02356-1
- Chiropractic-adjustments: verywellhealth.com, Retrieved 14 July, 2019
- Gorski, david (14 march 2011). “a university of michigan medical school alumnus confronts anthroposophic medicine at his alma mater”. Science-based medicine. Retrieved 29 november 2018

PERMISSIONS

All chapters in this book are published with permission under the Creative Commons Attribution Share Alike License or equivalent. Every chapter published in this book has been scrutinized by our experts. Their significance has been extensively debated. The topics covered herein carry significant information for a comprehensive understanding. They may even be implemented as practical applications or may be referred to as a beginning point for further studies.

We would like to thank the editorial team for lending their expertise to make the book truly unique. They have played a crucial role in the development of this book. Without their invaluable contributions this book wouldn't have been possible. They have made vital efforts to compile up to date information on the varied aspects of this subject to make this book a valuable addition to the collection of many professionals and students.

This book was conceptualized with the vision of imparting up-to-date and integrated information in this field. To ensure the same, a matchless editorial board was set up. Every individual on the board went through rigorous rounds of assessment to prove their worth. After which they invested a large part of their time researching and compiling the most relevant data for our readers.

The editorial board has been involved in producing this book since its inception. They have spent rigorous hours researching and exploring the diverse topics which have resulted in the successful publishing of this book. They have passed on their knowledge of decades through this book. To expedite this challenging task, the publisher supported the team at every step. A small team of assistant editors was also appointed to further simplify the editing procedure and attain best results for the readers.

Apart from the editorial board, the designing team has also invested a significant amount of their time in understanding the subject and creating the most relevant covers. They scrutinized every image to scout for the most suitable representation of the subject and create an appropriate cover for the book.

The publishing team has been an ardent support to the editorial, designing and production team. Their endless efforts to recruit the best for this project, has resulted in the accomplishment of this book. They are a veteran in the field of academics and their pool of knowledge is as vast as their experience in printing. Their expertise and guidance has proved useful at every step. Their uncompromising quality standards have made this book an exceptional effort. Their encouragement from time to time has been an inspiration for everyone.

The publisher and the editorial board hope that this book will prove to be a valuable piece of knowledge for students, practitioners and scholars across the globe.

INDEX

www.ingramcontent.com/pod-product-compliance
Lightning Source LLC
LaVergne TN
LVHW062128200926
848484LV00007B/1784
* 9 7 8 1 6 4 7 4 0 1 0 4 7 *